Albert Kikonzi

Zoonoses and public health

Albert Kikonzi

Zoonoses and public health

Prevention and control approaches

ScienciaScripts

Imprint

Cover image: www.ingimage.com

This book is a translation from the original published under ISBN 978-620-6-72849-8.

Publisher:
Sciencia Scripts
is a trademark of
Dodo Books Indian Ocean Ltd. and OmniScriptum S.R.L publishing group

120 High Road, East Finchley, London, N2 9ED, United Kingdom
Str. Armeneasca 28/1, office 1, Chisinau MD-2012, Republic of Moldova, Europe
Printed at: see last page
ISBN: 978-620-8-34768-0

Foreword

In an increasingly interconnected world, zoonoses - diseases transmissible between animals and humans - represent a major public health challenge. The rise in international trade, increasing urbanization and climate change have created fertile ground for the emergence and re-emergence of these infections. This book, which aims to explore the vast field of zoonoses, is intended as a valuable resource for health professionals, researchers and the general public.

Zoonoses are not just exotic diseases; they affect millions of people worldwide. From well-known infections such as rabies, M-pox, covid-19, tuberculosis and leptospirosis to less familiar pathologies such as schistosomiasis and filariasis, their impact on human health is considerable. Understanding transmission mechanisms, risk factors and prevention strategies is essential if we are to combat these diseases effectively.

This book is structured around several chapters, each dedicated to a specific zoonosis, while integrating perspectives on global health. We address the ethical, economic and environmental issues associated with these infections, as well as the multidisciplinary approaches needed to combat them. Case studies will illustrate the challenges faced in different parts of the world, highlighting efforts to control and prevent zoonoses. We hope that this book will inspire not only industry professionals, but also decision-makers, students and anyone concerned with human and animal health. Ultimately, the fight against zoonoses requires close cooperation between disciplines, nations and communities.

We hope this book will help to raise awareness, inform, and mobilize the efforts needed to tackle this critically important public health issue.

Professor LUTONADJO

Dedication

To my parents,
for their unfailing support and unconditional love,
who taught me the importance of curiosity and compassion.

To my mentors, for their wise counsel and inspiration,
who have guided my path in the quest for knowledge.

To all the healthcare professionals and researchers whose dedication and passion make a difference every day,
and who work tirelessly for a healthier world.

To my darling Maguy, my children whom I love dearly: Princesse KIKONZI AND Gradie KIKONZI.

To my big brothers whom I love dearly, Abbé KIKONZI, CT willy KIKONZI MATINA and my only sister Godélive KIKONZI.

To Papa Pasteur **MABAYA Jean-Pierre** and all his family,

To all my nephews and nieces, Borel KIBALA, Jeancy KIBALA, Bénédicte KIBALA, Jackson KIBALA and Sarah KIBALA, Jeancy KIKONZI, Christopher KIKONZI, Mbo and Mpia KIKONZI, Winnette and Judelle KIKONZI

To my uncles, Matthieu NDUKUTE, Bizen NDUKUTE, Siros BATETE

To my brothers and friends Joël KASUKASU, Delphin MUSESE, Marcel LUBALA, Ali KISUPA, Emmanuel NYOGA, Maître Urbain KAMWANGA, assistant Hugues DIOSI, IKUMA Patrick and others.

To my old CT martin NYOGA and his wife Madame CT J'acquis.

To the entire ISP MUKEDI scientific family

To all those working for a healthier world, may this book be a source of inspiration and commitment as we work together to meet the challenges of public health.

Finally, to all those affected by zoonoses, in the hope that this book will help raise awareness and provide solutions.

I dedicate this book

Dr. Albert KIKONZI PROJECT MANAGER

Thanks

I would like to express my deep gratitude to all those who have contributed to the production of this book.

First of all, a huge thank you to my parents, whose constant support and encouragement have enabled me to pursue my dreams and bring this project to fruition. Their faith in me has been an invaluable source of motivation.

I would also like to thank my mentors and colleagues, whose advice and expertise have been invaluable throughout my research. You shared your knowledge generously, and your passion for research and public health was an inspiration. Thank you all so much.

A special thanks to the Director General of ISP MUKEDI Professor **Albert GAPINGA**, to the Secretary General **CT KAFUTI, to** the scientific body of ISP MUKEDI and to the research team who collaborated with me, bringing innovative ideas and enriching perspectives. Your hard work and dedication have greatly contributed to the quality of this book.

I would also like to thank the health professionals and researchers who, through their daily efforts, face up to the challenges of zoonoses. Your commitment to the well-being of our communities is admirable and essential.

Finally, thanks to my friends, brothers and elders, Fabrice NDUKU, Etienne KITOKO, CT André ILUNGA, Daniel MIKULU, Julien Mbwamulungu, Dr. Felix MATIALA, Assistant LUBALA Marcel, Jean Paul KASANJI, Assistant Jean-Claude MUNZUMBU, **Abbé KIVUDI,** Abbé Jean - Remy yamvwa, CT LUNGOY, CT Caroline SANDUKU for their unconditional support and for believing in me, even in moments of doubt.

I dedicate this work to all of you, in the hope that it will raise awareness and provide solutions to the public health issues that concern us all.

CT. Dr. Albert KIKONZI

Introduction

Zoonoses are infectious diseases transmissible from animals to humans, and represent a major challenge for global public health. With human population growth, increasing urbanization and climate change, interactions between humans and animals are multiplying, favoring the emergence and spread of these diseases. Historically, zoonoses have played a significant role in the evolution of human societies, influencing events such as devastating epidemics and changes in agricultural practices.

Understanding zoonoses is essential not only for the protection of human health, but also for the preservation of animal health and the environment. Zoonoses represent a complex link between animal health, human health and the ecosystem as a whole, illustrating the concept of "One Health". This principle underlines the interdependence of animal, human and environmental health systems, and highlights the need for collaborative approaches to combating these diseases.[1]

The aim of this book is to explore the public health dimensions of zoonoses. It will cover the main zoonoses, their impact on human and animal health, and approaches to prevention and control. By examining the challenges, opportunities and innovations in this field, we hope to provide a valuable resource for health professionals, decision-makers and anyone interested in public health and health risk management.

Through an in-depth analysis of zoonoses, this book aims to raise awareness of the importance of an integrated, proactive response, ensuring better protection against the threats these diseases pose to our collective health.[2]

---

[1] Acha P.N., Szyfres B., 2005. *Zoonoses and communicable diseases common to man and animals*, OIE.

[2] Artaud H. *et al.*, 2019. *Museum Manifesto. Humans and other animals.* Reliefs/MNHN, https://www.mnhn.fr/fr/explorez/actualites/ manifest-museum-humans-other-animals.

Definitions and significance of zoonoses

Definitions

The word "**zoonosis**" comes from the Greek roots *ζῷον (zôon*, animal) and *νόσος* (*nosos*, disease). As early as antiquity, the possibility of transmission of certain diseases from animals to humans was evoked, notably in the case of rabies, but it was in the 19th century that the concepts of microbes, contagion, infection and transmission appeared, at least in their contemporary senses, paving the way for microbiology and epidemiology.[3]

It was the German physician and researcher **Rudolph Virchow** (1821-1902) who coined the term zoonosis after noting the links between a parasitic disease present in pigs and humans, trichinellosis (see p. 92). Today, a zoonosis (or zoonotic disease) is defined as an infectious or parasitic disease whose microbial or parasitic agents are naturally transmitted between humans and animals.

Zoonoses are infectious diseases that can be transmitted from animals to humans and back again. This transmission can occur directly, through contact with infected animals or their excrement, or indirectly, via vectors such as insects, or through the environment. Zoonoses can be caused by a variety of pathogens, such as :

- **Viruses**: such as the rabies virus or the avian flu virus.
- **Bacteria**: such as *Salmonella* or *Leptospira*.
- **Parasites**: such as the protozoa responsible for toxoplasmosis.[4]

---

[3] Barnouin J., Sache Y., 2010. *Emerging diseases. Epidemiology in plants, animals and humans*. Editions Qu..

[4] Blanc S., Boetsch G., Hossaert-McKey M., Renaud F., 2017. *Health ecology*, https://www.cnrs.fr/fr/ecologie-de-la-sante-pour-unenouvelle-read-my-health.

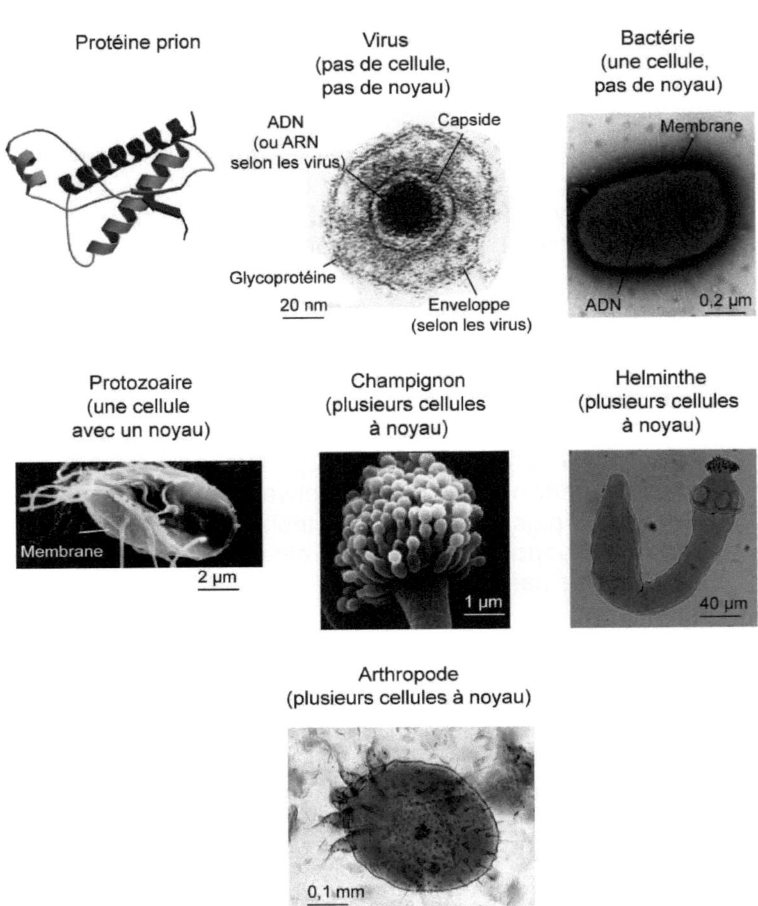

- Figure 1. Zoonotic agents.

What is Public Health?

Public health is a multidisciplinary field that focuses on protecting and improving the health of populations through organized, collective efforts. It aims to prevent disease, prolong life and promote health through collective action. Here are a few key points to help you better understand this concept.[5]

[5] Duvallet G., Fontenille D., Robert V., 2017. *Medical and veterinary entomology*. IRD Editions, Editions Qu..

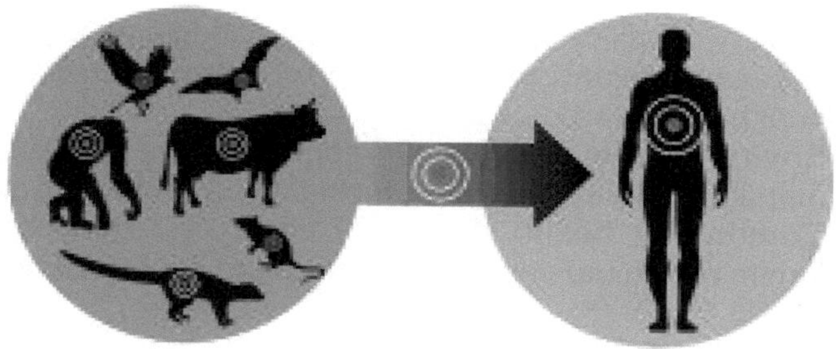

Chez les humains, les zoonoses représentent
60 % de **toutes les maladies infectieuses** et
75 % des maladies infectieuses **émergentes.**

***Source** : d'après le rapport Frontières 2016 du PNUE*

Figure 2: Accessed on October 30, 2024 at 7:03 pm

1. Definition and objectives

- **Definition**: Public health encompasses all the activities and policies implemented to protect and improve the health of populations. This includes disease surveillance, health promotion, disease prevention and health crisis management.
- **Objectives** : The main objectives of public health are:
  - Prevent illness and injury.
  - Promoting healthy lifestyles.
  - Improving access to healthcare.
  - Responding to health crises.[6]

2. Areas of intervention

Public health encompasses several areas, including :

- **Epidemiology**: Study of the distribution and determinants of disease in populations.

[6] Guegan J.-F., Choisy M., 2008. *Introduction to the integrative epidemiology of infectious and parasitic diseases*. De Boeck Super eur.

- **Health promotion**: Initiatives designed to encourage healthy behavior and improve living conditions.
- **Disease prevention**: Vaccination programs, screening and health risk awareness.
- **Environmental health**: Protecting human health by managing the environment, including air and water quality.
- **Community health**: Initiatives designed to improve the health of communities through targeted interventions.[7]

3. Methods and strategies

- **Surveillance and Research**: collecting data on the health of populations to identify health problems and assess the effectiveness of interventions.
- **Health policies**: drafting laws and regulations to protect public health (e.g. banning smoking in public places).
- **Education and Awareness**: Information programs to raise public awareness of health issues, such as nutrition and disease prevention.
- **Community interventions**: projects and programs carried out at local level to meet the specific needs of local populations.

4. Importance of Public Health

- **Disease prevention** : Public health is essential to prevent epidemics and chronic diseases, thus contributing to longevity and quality of life.
- **Health Equity**: Aims to reduce health inequalities by tackling the social determinants of health.[8]
- **Crisis management**: In times of health crisis, such as a pandemic, public health plays a crucial role in coordinating responses and protecting populations.

Public health is a vital field that seeks to improve the health of populations through coordinated, evidence-based action. By tackling the determinants of health and

[7] Leport C., Guegan J.-F., 2011. *Emerging infectious diseases: status and outlook*. La Documentation française, https://www. Vie publique.fr/rapport/31962-les-maladies-infectieuses-emergentesetat- de-la-situation et-perspecti.

[8]

promoting healthy behaviors, public health contributes to the creation of healthier, more resilient societies.

Importance of Zoonoses

1. **Public health**: Zoonoses represent a significant threat to human health. Diseases such as avian influenza, rabies and Lyme disease have a considerable impact on morbidity and mortality worldwide. Understanding and controlling these diseases is therefore essential to protect public health.[9]
2. **Economy**: Zoonoses can have severe economic consequences, affecting the agricultural and livestock sectors. Epidemics can result in significant financial losses due to reduced animal productivity, healthcare costs and the control measures required to limit the spread of disease.
3. **Food safety**: Zoonoses can contaminate the food chain, putting food safety at risk. Food-borne infections, often caused by zoonotic pathogens, can lead to epidemics of gastroenteritis and other food-borne illnesses.
4. **Ecosystems**: Zoonoses are also an indicator of ecosystem health. Deforestation, urbanization and climate change are altering natural habitats, increasing human-wildlife interactions and facilitating disease transmission.
5. **Research and development**: The study of zoonoses stimulates research in various fields, such as microbiology, epidemiology and veterinary medicine. Discoveries in this field can lead to innovations in diagnosis, treatment and prevention strategies.

In summary, we need to be aware that zoonoses are a major issue affecting many aspects of our society. Understanding and managing them is crucial to promoting human, animal and environmental health, and to ensuring a healthier, more sustainable future for all.[10]

---

[9] Report by the Foundation for Biodiversity Research (FRB), 2020. *Mobilisation de la FRB par les pouvoirs publics français sur les liens entre Covid-19 et biodiversité*,https://www.fondationbiodiversite.fr/wp-content/uploads/2020/05/Mobilisation-FRBCovid- 19-15-05-2020-1.pdf.

[10] Report of the "Intergovernmental Science-Policy Platform on Biodiversity and Ecosystem Services" (IPBES) seminar on Escaping the Era of

Zoonosis Prevention and Control

Preventing and controlling zoonoses requires an integrated approach combining public health, animal health and environmental protection strategies. [2]The key measures for preventing and controlling zoonoses are :

1. Monitoring and Detection

- **Surveillance systems**: Set up epidemiological surveillance systems for the early detection of zoonoses in animals and humans. This includes collecting data on suspected cases and outbreaks.
- **Reporting and Information Sharing**: Encourage information sharing between human, animal and environmental health sectors for rapid response.

2. Vaccination

- **Animal Vaccination**: Develop and promote vaccination programs for domestic animals (such as dogs and cats) and farm animals to reduce the risk of transmission to humans.[11]
- **Awareness campaigns**: Inform pet owners about the importance of vaccination to protect public and animal health.

3. Food hygiene and safety

- **Hygiene practices**: Promote proper hygiene practices when handling, preparing and consuming food of animal origin.
- **Food Chain Control**: Implement strict regulations on food production, storage and distribution to prevent contamination by zoonotic pathogens.

4. Education and awareness

Pandemics, 2020, https://ipbes.net/pandemics. Vittecoq M., Roche B., Prugnolle F., Renaud F., Thomas F., 2015. *Les maladies infectieuses*. De Boeck-Solal.

[11] Morand S., 2016. *The next plague. A global history of societies and their epidemics.* Editions Fayard.

- **Education programs**: Develop educational programs for communities on zoonoses, their modes of transmission and preventive measures.
- **Community involvement**: Involving communities in public health initiatives such as vaccination campaigns and clean-up days.

5. Animal and Environmental Management

- **Animal population control**: Set up programs to manage animal populations, particularly wild animals and rodents, which can act as reservoirs for zoonoses.
- **Environmental protection**: Promote sustainable agricultural practices and environmental conservation policies to reduce the risk of zoonosis transmission.[12]

6. Intersectoral collaboration

- **One Health approach**: Adopt a One Health approach that integrates the efforts of the human, animal and environmental health sectors for a coordinated response to zoonoses.
- **Partnerships**: Establish partnerships between governments, NGOs, researchers and communities to share resources and information.[13]

7. Research & Innovation

- **Investing in research**: Support research into zoonotic pathogens, including their transmission, evolution and best prevention practices.
- **Development of New Tools**: Encourage the development of new technologies for the rapid diagnosis, vaccination and treatment of zoonoses.
-

- **Who's concerned?**

In local authorities, the professional activities concerned by zoonoses are very diverse, for example :

---

[12] Morand S., 2020. *Man, wildlife and the plague.* Editions Fayard.

[13] Morand S., Figuie M., 2016. *Emerging infectious diseases. Risques et enjeux de société.* Editions Qu..

- Environmental jobs such as wastewater collection and treatment, waste collection and treatment, maintenance of voluntary drop-off points or waste collection centers, deratting, river and canal bank maintenance;
- Forestry jobs such as lumberjack or nature warden;
- Activities involving contact with animals, impounding or capturing stray animals
- Dead animal collection and rendering;
- Taxidermy...
- Other professions may also be affected, particularly when working in high-risk areas or on high-risk sites. For example, an electrician working in a rodent-infested crawl space.[14]

Preventing and controlling zoonoses requires an integrated, collaborative approach. By strengthening surveillance, improving hygiene practices, educating communities and adopting a One Health approach, it is possible to effectively reduce the risk of zoonoses and protect public health. Cooperation between sectors is essential to create resilient and responsive health systems in the face of zoonotic threats.[15]

Objectives

This book aims to achieve several key objectives to better understand and address the issue of zoonoses in the context of public health:

1. **Educate and raise awareness**: To provide an in-depth understanding of zoonoses, including their definition, classification and impact on human and animal health. The book aims to make the public, decision-makers and healthcare professionals aware of the importance of this issue.
2. **Analyze public health issues**: Highlight the public health challenges posed by zoonoses, including past

[14] Morand S., Lajaunie C., 2018. *Biodiversity and health. Links between living organisms, ecosystems and societies.* ISTE/Elsevier.

[15] Morand S., Moutou F., Richomme C., 2014. *Faune sauvage, biodiversité et santé, quels défis?* Editions Qu..

epidemics and their consequences, to better prepare healthcare systems to deal with these threats.

3. **Exploring risk factors**: Identify and examine the environmental, societal and behavioral factors that contribute to the emergence and spread of zoonoses. This includes interactions between humans, animals and their environment.

4. **Present prevention and control strategies**: Propose evidence-based approaches to the prevention and control of zoonoses. This includes recommendations on vaccination, hygiene, surveillance and risk management.

5. **Promoting the One Health approach**: Emphasizing the importance of interdisciplinary collaboration between the human, animal and environmental health sectors. The book will encourage an integrated vision, essential for an effective response to zoonoses.

6. **Provide case studies**: Illustrate theoretical concepts with concrete examples of zoonotic disease outbreaks, highlighting lessons learned and best practices in public health management.

7. **Encourage research and innovation**: Stimulate interest in research into zoonoses and their management, highlighting technological and methodological innovations likely to improve the detection, prevention and treatment of these diseases.

8. **Assessing future prospects**: Analyze emerging trends in zoonoses and discuss future implications for public health, taking into account environmental, social and economic changes.

In short, this book aspires to be a valuable resource for researchers, health professionals, decision-makers and anyone involved in the fight against zoonoses, promoting collective understanding and action in the face of this complex, multidimensional issue.

Current Zoonoses and Public Health Context

Emergence and re-emergence of zoonoses

In recent decades, we have witnessed a significant increase in emerging and re-emerging zoonoses. Diseases such as Ebola, Zika virus, and more recently SARS-CoV-2, have demonstrated how zoonoses can cross the species barrier and cause global pandemics. This trend is exacerbated by the intensification of human activities, such as rapid urbanization, deforestation, and climate change, which are altering animals' natural habitats and increasing human-animal interactions.[16]

Impact of climate change

Climate change plays a crucial role in the dynamics of zoonoses. Changes in temperature, precipitation and ecosystems can favor the spread of certain diseases. For example, vectors such as mosquitoes, which transmit diseases such as malaria and dengue fever, may extend their geographical range as a result of global warming. In addition, extreme climatic events, such as floods and droughts, can disrupt health systems and increase the risk of zoonosis transmission.

Globalization and Mobility

Globalization has facilitated the mobility of people and goods, increasing the risk of zoonoses spreading rapidly. The international transport of animals and food products, combined with frequent travel, enables pathogens to spread from one region to another in record time. The recent COVID-19 pandemic has highlighted this vulnerability, underscoring the need for increased international public health surveillance and cooperation.[17]

Public Health and Health Systems

Public health systems face increasing challenges in detecting, monitoring and controlling zoonoses. The need for an integrated approach, linking human, animal and environmental health sectors, is more pressing than ever. One Health" initiatives are essential to improve

---

[16] Moutou F., 2020. *Epidemics, animals and people.* Editions Le Pommier.

[17]

World Health Organization (WHO). WHO | Zoonoses and the Environment [Internet]. WHO. World Health Organization; 2020 [cited26 Apr2020]. Available from: https://www.who.int/foodsafety/areas_work/zoonose/fr/

collaboration between different disciplines and ensure a coordinated response to health threats.

Awareness and Education

Public awareness and education about zoonoses are crucial to preventing their spread. Human behavior, such as eating wild animals or failing to observe hygiene measures, can exacerbate the risk of transmission. Educational programs and awareness campaigns are therefore essential to encourage safer practices.

The current zoonoses and public health context is marked by a convergence of complex, interconnected factors that require urgent attention and collective action. To meet these challenges, it is imperative to adopt integrated approaches and strengthen collaboration between the health, environment and agriculture sectors, in order to protect the health of human and animal populations in a constantly changing world.

Key facts

- A zoonosis is a disease or infection naturally transmissible from vertebrate animals to humans.
- There are over 200 known types of zoonosis.
- Zoonoses account for a large percentage of new and existing human diseases.
- Some zoonoses, such as rabies, are completely preventable by vaccination or other methods.

A zoonosis is an infectious disease that has been transmitted from animals to humans. Zoonotic pathogens may be bacterial, viral or parasitic in origin, or may involve non-conventional agents and spread to humans through direct contact or via food, water or the environment. They represent a major public health problem worldwide, due to our close relationship with animals in various contexts (agriculture, domestic animals and the natural environment). Zoonoses can also disrupt the production and trade of products of animal origin for food or other purposes.

Zoonoses account for a large proportion of all newly identified infectious diseases, as well as many existing ones. Some diseases, such as HIV, begin as zoonoses, but later mutate into strains found only in humans.[18] Other zoonoses can cause recurrent outbreaks, such as Ebola virus disease and salmonellosis. Still others, like the new coronavirus behind COVID-19, have the potential to cause global pandemics.

Prevention and control

Zoonosis prevention methods differ for each pathogen; however, several practices are recognized as effective in reducing risks at community and personal levels. Safe and appropriate animal care guidelines in the agricultural sector reduce the risk of food-borne zoonosis outbreaks via foods such as meat, eggs, dairy products or even certain vegetables.[19] Standards for drinking water and waste disposal, as well as the protection of surface water in the natural environment, are also important and effective. Information campaigns to promote hand-washing after contact with animals and other behavioral adjustments help to reduce the community spread of zoonoses when they do occur.

Antimicrobial resistance is a further complicating factor in the fight against zoonoses. The widespread use of antibiotics in food-producing animals increases the risk of drug-resistant strains of zoonotic pathogens that can spread rapidly to animals and humans.

---

[18] HubálekZ. Emerging Human Infectious Diseases: Anthroponoses, Zoonoses, and Sapronoses-Volume 9, Number 3-March 2003 -Emerging Infectious Diseases journal CDC. 2003 [cited26 Apr2020];9(3). Available from: https://wwwnc.cdc.gov/eid/article/9/3/02-0208_article

[19] Lowe A-M. Bulletin de l'Observatoire multipartite québécois sur les zoonoses et l'adaptation aux changements climatiques, Volume1, Issue 1 [Internet]. INSPQ. [cited 26 Apr2020]. Available from: https://www.inspq.qc.ca/bulletin-de-l-observatoire-multipartite-quebecois-sur-les-zoonoses-et-l-adaptation-aux-changements-climatiques/janvier-2016

Who is at risk?

Zoonotic pathogens can spread to humans through any point of contact with domestic, agricultural or wild animals. Markets selling wild animal meat or by-products present a particularly high risk, due to the high number of new or unrecorded pathogens known to exist in certain wild animal populations. Farm workers in areas where antibiotics are heavily administered to farm animals may be exposed to an increased risk of pathogens resistant to current antimicrobial drugs. People living near wilderness areas, or in semi-urban areas where the number of wild animals is higher, are at risk of contracting diseases transmitted by animals such as rats, foxes or raccoons. Urbanization and the destruction of natural habitats increase the risk of zoonoses by increasing contact between humans and wild animals.

WHO action

WHO collaborates with national governments, universities, non-governmental organizations, philanthropic bodies and regional and international partners to prevent and manage zoonotic threats and their impact on public health, social and economic consequences. These efforts include the promotion of intersectoral collaboration at the human-animal-environment interface between the different sectors concerned at regional, national and international levels.[20] WHO also strives to build capacity and promote practical, evidence-based and cost-effective tools and mechanisms for the prevention, monitoring and detection of zoonoses through reporting, epidemiological and laboratory investigation, risk assessment and control, and to support countries in implementation.[21]

As part of the "One World, One Health" approach, the World Health Organization is collaborating with the Food and Agriculture Organization of the United Nations (FAO)

[20] Larousse É. Definitions: prion -Dictionnaire de français Larousse [Internet]. [cited 26 Apr2020]. Available from: https://www.larousse.fr/dictionnaires/francais/prion/63977

[21] PrusinerSB. Novelproteinaceousinfectiousparticlescause scrapie. Science. 9 avr1982;216(4542):136-44.

and the World Organization for Animal Health (OIE) on the Global Animal Disease Early Warning and Response System. This joint system capitalizes on the added value of combining and coordinating the alert mechanisms of the three organizations to support early warning, prevention and control of animal disease threats, including zoonoses, through data exchange and risk assessment.

Ecology and Zoonoses: A Complex Relationship

1. Introduction

Ecology plays a fundamental role in the dynamics of zoonoses, the transmissible diseases between animals and humans. Understanding this relationship is essential to developing effective prevention and control strategies.

2. Ecological interactions

a. Biodiversity and Zoonoses

- **Role of Biodiversity**: High biodiversity can reduce the risk of zoonoses by maintaining healthy ecosystems. Diverse animal populations can limit pathogen transmission by diluting interactions between host species and pathogens.[22]
- **Effect of Species Extinction**: The loss of biodiversity, often caused by human activity, can increase the risk of zoonoses. For example, the reduction of natural predators can favor populations of vector animals, such as rodents.

b. Habitat changes

- **Urbanization**: The expansion of urban areas encroaches on natural habitats, which can lead to increased contact between humans and wild animals, increasing the risk of disease transmission.

---

[22] Larousse É. Definitions: parasite -Dictionnaire de français Larousse [Internet]. [cited 26 Apr2020]. Available from: https://www.larousse.fr/dictionnaires/francais/parasite/58023

- **Deforestation**: The destruction of forests for agriculture or logging can disrupt ecosystems and force animals closer to inhabited areas, increasing the risk of infection.

3. Climate change

- **Impact on vectors**: Climate change can alter the geographical distribution of vectors such as mosquitoes and ticks, increasing the risk of zoonotic epidemics in new regions.
- **Pathogen adaptation**: Pathogens themselves can evolve and adapt to new environmental conditions, making certain zoonoses more difficult to control.

4. Agriculture & Livestock

- **Farming practices**: Intensive livestock farming and industrial agriculture can create conditions conducive to the emergence of zoonoses, by encouraging the spread of disease between animals.
- **Antibiotic use**: Overuse of antibiotics in livestock farming can lead to antimicrobial resistance, making infections more difficult to treat.

5. Ecological monitoring

- **Disease surveillance** : Monitoring ecosystems and animal populations is essential for early detection of zoonoses. Integrated surveillance systems can help identify potential risks before they become epidemics.
- **Ecosystem approaches**: Integrating ecologically-based approaches into public and animal health management can improve the effectiveness of interventions.

Worth knowing:

The relationship between ecology and zoonoses is complex and multidimensional. Protecting biodiversity, managing habitats sustainably, and integrating ecological approaches into public health are essential to reduce the risk of zoonoses emerging. By adopting a "One Health" perspective, linking human, animal and environmental health, we can better anticipate and manage the challenges posed by zoonoses in a constantly changing world.

CHAPTER 1: UNDERSTANDING ZOONOSES

1.1. Definition and Classification of Zoonoses

1.1.1. Definition of Zoonoses

Zoonoses are infectious diseases that can be transmitted from animals to humans. This transmission can occur in various ways, including :

- **Direct transmission**: Contamination through direct contact with infected animals, their body fluids or feces.[23]
- **Indirect transmission**: Transmission via vectors (such as mosquitoes or ticks) or the environment (contaminated water, soil, food).

Zoonoses can be caused by a variety of pathogens, including viruses, bacteria, parasites and fungi.[24]

1.1.2. Zoonoses classification

Zoonoses can be classified according to several criteria, including the type of pathogen, the mode of transmission and the severity of the disease. Here's an overview of the different classifications:

1.1.2.1. By pathogen

- **Viral zoonoses** :
  - Examples: rabies, avian flu, Ebola virus, Zika virus, covid-19, M-pox, Yellow Fever virus and others.
- **Bacterial zoonoses** :
  - Examples: leptospirosis, salmonellosis, tularemia, brucellosis, tuberculosis
- **Parasitic zoonoses** :
  - Examples: toxoplasmosis, Chagas disease, echinococcosis.

---

[23] BourgeadeA, DavoustB, GallaisH. FROM ANIMAL DISEASES TO HUMAN INFECTIONS. Médecine d'Afrique Noire. 1992;39(3):6.

[24] Larousse É. Definitions: parasite -Dictionnaire de français Larousse [Internet]. [cited 26 Apr2020]. Available from: https://www.larousse.fr/dictionnaires/francais/parasite/58023

- **Fungal zoonoses** :
  - Examples: histoplasmosis, cryptococcosis.
  -
  -
- **Viral zoonoses** :

Rabies

Rage: Overview and Key Aspects

1. What is Rabies?

Rabies is a serious viral disease that affects the central nervous system. It is caused by the rabies virus, a lyssavirus, and is transmitted mainly through the bite of an infected animal. Rabies is almost always fatal once symptoms appear, but is entirely preventable through vaccination.

2. Transmission

- **Main Vector**: Rabies is spread mainly by the saliva of infected animals, including dogs, bats, foxes and raccoons.
- **Mode of transmission**: Transmission usually occurs through biting, but can also occur through scratches or open wounds in contact with the saliva of an infected animal.

3. Symptoms

The symptoms of rabies can be classified into several phases:

- **Prodromal phase**: Initial symptoms include fever, headache, fatigue and a tingling or itching sensation at the bite site.
- **Aggressive phase**: This phase is characterized by neurological disorders such as anxiety, confusion, hallucinations, convulsions and swallowing disorders (hydrophobia).
- **Terminal phase**: Left untreated, rabies leads to paralysis, coma and finally death, usually by respiratory arrest.

4. Prevention

- **Vaccinating pets**: Vaccinating pets, especially dogs, is one of the most effective ways of preventing rabies.
- **Preventive vaccination**: People at risk (healthcare workers, veterinarians, etc.) can receive preventive vaccinations.
- **Education and awareness**: Inform people about the dangers of rabies and the importance of reporting animal bites.

5. Treatment

- **Post-exposure**: If a person is bitten by an animal suspected of being rabid, he or she should immediately consult a healthcare professional. Post-exposure treatment, including injections of rabies vaccine and immunoglobulin, is essential to prevent the onset of the disease.
- **No Curative Treatment**: Once the symptoms of rabies appear, there is no effective treatment, and the disease is usually fatal.[25]

6. Global Impact

- **Statistics**: According to the World Health Organization (WHO), rabies causes around 59,000 deaths a year worldwide, mainly in developing countries where animal vaccination is inadequate.
- **Areas at risk**: Rabies-endemic regions include parts of Africa, Asia and Latin America.[26]

Rabies is a preventable disease, but it remains a major public health problem in many parts of the world. Animal vaccination, public education and effective treatment measures can significantly reduce the risk of infection and protect communities. An integrated approach involving

---

[25] Zoonotic Diseases | One Health | CDC [Internet]. 2020 [cited 26 Apr2020]. Available from: https://www.cdc.gov/onehealth/basics/zoonotic-diseases.html

[26] World Organisation for Animal Health (OIE). One health: OIE -World Organisation for Animal Health [Internet]. 2020 [cited 26 Apr2020]. Available from: https://www.oie.int/fr/pour-les-medias/une-seule-sante/

animal and public health is essential to eradicate this disease.

Avian Influenza: Overview and Key Aspects

1. What is Avian Influenza?

Avian influenza, also known as bird flu, is a viral infection that mainly affects birds, but can also infect other species, including humans. It is caused by viruses of the Orthomyxoviridae family, mainly subtypes H5 and H7, which can be highly pathogenic.

2. Transmission

- **Between birds**: Avian flu is spread mainly between birds by direct contact with infected birds, their droppings, or contaminated surfaces.
- **Transmission to humans**: Human infections are rare and usually occur after close contact with infected birds or their environments. Human-to-human transmission is extremely rare.

3. Symptoms

a. In birds

- **Symptoms**: Symptoms may vary depending on the virulence of the virus, ranging from mild to severe, including :
  - Depression and apathy
  - Breathing difficulties
  - Reduced egg-laying products
  - High mortality for highly pathogenic strains

b. In humans

- **Symptoms**: When infected, humans may experience symptoms similar to those of seasonal flu, such as :
  - Fever
  - Cough
  - Sore throats
  - Myalgias

- **Complications**: In severe cases, this can lead to pneumonia and potentially fatal respiratory complications.

4. Prevention

- **Avian surveillance**: Set up surveillance programs to detect avian influenza strains in domestic and wild birds.
- **Farm control**: Apply strict biosecurity measures on poultry farms to prevent the introduction and spread of the virus.
- **Vaccination**: Vaccinating poultry in high-risk areas can help control the spread of the virus.

5. Control and processing

- **Epidemic response**: When a highly pathogenic strain is detected, it is often necessary to cull infected poultry to limit spread.
- **Human treatment**: Antivirals such as oseltamivir (Tamiflu) can be effective if administered early after exposure to the virus.

6. Global Impact

- **Epidemics**: Avian flu has caused several large-scale epidemics, affecting bird populations and leading to significant economic losses in the poultry industry.
- **Public health**: Although human transmission is rare, cases of avian flu in humans raise concerns about the possibility of a pandemic if the virus acquires the ability to transmit efficiently between humans.

Avian influenza represents a significant challenge to animal and public health. Surveillance, prevention and outbreak control are essential to minimize the impact of this disease. Collaboration between the animal and human health sectors, as well as effective communication, are crucial to managing the risks associated with avian flu.

Ebola Virus: Overview and Key Aspects

1. What is the Ebola Virus?

The Ebola virus is a highly virulent pathogen responsible for Ebola hemorrhagic fever (EHF). It belongs to the

Filoviridae family and is characterized by high mortality rates, reaching up to 90% in certain epidemics.[27] The virus was first identified in 1976 during epidemics in the Democratic Republic of Congo (DRC) and Sudan.

2. Transmission

- **Human transmission**: The Ebola virus is spread mainly by direct contact with the bodily fluids of an infected person (blood, saliva, sweat, vomit, etc.) or by contact with contaminated objects.[28]
- **Animal reservoir**: Fruit bats are considered the natural reservoir of the virus. Initial transmission to humans may occur through hunting or consumption of infected wild animals, such as monkeys or antelopes.

3. Symptoms

Symptoms of Ebola virus infection usually appear between 2 and 21 days after exposure and include:

- **Initial phase** :
  - Fever
  - Headache
  - Muscle pain
  - Fatigue
- **Advanced phase** :
  - Vomiting
  - Diarrhea
  - Skin rashes
  - Internal and external bleeding (in severe cases)

4. Prevention

[27] One Health initiative. One Health Initiative -One World One Medicine One Health [Internet]. Mission Statement. [cited 26 Apr2020]. Available from: http://www.onehealthinitiative.com/mission.php

[28] Han BA, Kramer AM, Drake JM. Global Patterns of Zoonotic Disease in Mammals. Trends in Parasitology. 1 Jul 2016 ;32(7) :565-77.

- **Epidemic control**: Public health measures such as surveillance, case isolation and contact management are crucial to controlling epidemics.
- **Training and awareness**: Educate communities about modes of transmission and prevention behaviors, such as avoiding contact with bodily fluids.
- **Vaccination**: The rVSV-ZEBOV vaccine, developed against the Ebola virus, has proved effective and is used in vaccination campaigns during epidemics.
-

5. Treatment

- **Supportive care**: There is no specific antiviral treatment for Ebola, but supportive care, such as rehydration, symptom management and treatment of secondary infections, is essential to improve chances of survival.
- **Antivirals**: Experimental treatments have been used in certain situations and show promise.

6. Global Impact

- **Epidemics**: Ebola epidemics have mainly affected countries in West and Central Africa, with a major outbreak in 2014-2016 affecting several countries, including Guinea, Liberia and Sierra Leone, causing more than 11,000 deaths.[29]
- **Health concerns**: The highly contagious and deadly nature of the Ebola virus makes it a global public health threat, requiring continuous vigilance and response capabilities.

We need to be aware that the Ebola virus represents a major public health challenge, due to its virulence and transmission potential. Epidemic prevention relies on appropriate surveillance, education, vaccination and care strategies. International collaboration is essential to control epidemics and protect vulnerable communities. Lessons

---

[29] Van den Berg T. One health paradigm to foster population health [Internet]. BiomedCentral. 2020 [cited 26 Apr2020]. Available from: https://www.biomedcentral.com/collections/OneHealth

from past epidemics have led to improvements in preparedness and response to Ebola-related health crises.

Zika virus: Overview and key aspects

1. What is the Zika Virus?

The Zika virus is a flavivirus transmitted mainly by mosquitoes, notably **Aedes aegypti** and **Aedes albopictus**. First identified in 1947 in Uganda, it has since caused epidemics in various regions, notably Latin America and the Caribbean.

2. Transmission

- **Vector transmission**: The virus is spread mainly by the bites of infected mosquitoes.
- **Human transmission**: It can also be transmitted by :
  - Sexual contact with an infected person.
  - Transmission from mother to child during pregnancy or childbirth.
  - Blood transfusions.

3. Symptoms

Symptoms of Zika virus infection are generally mild and may include:

- Mild fever
- Skin rashes
- Joint and muscle pain
- Conjunctivitis (redness of the eyes)
- Headache

Symptoms generally appear between 2 and 7 days after the bite of an infected mosquito, and last about a week.

4. Complications

- **Microcephaly**: One of the most serious complications associated with Zika virus infection during pregnancy is microcephaly, a congenital malformation characterized by abnormal development of the fetal skull and brain.

- **Guillain-Barré syndrome**: Zika virus infection has also been linked to an increased risk of Guillain-Barré syndrome, an autoimmune disease that can lead to muscle weakness and paralysis.

5. Prevention

- **Mosquito control**: Eliminate mosquito breeding areas, such as containers of stagnant water, and use insecticides.
- **Personal protection**: Wear long clothing, use repellents containing DEET, and install mosquito nets to protect against bites.
- **Education**: Raising community awareness of transmission risks and preventive measures.

6. Treatment

There is no specific antiviral treatment for Zika virus. Management focuses on symptom relief, including:

- Rest
- Hydration
- Analgesics (such as paracetamol)

7. Global Impact

- **Epidemics**: The Zika virus has caused notable epidemics, particularly in 2015-2016, when the virus rapidly circulated in the Americas, causing major concerns about birth defects.
- **Surveillance and research**: The situation has led to increased surveillance and research efforts to better understand the virus, its modes of transmission and its effects on health.

To remember: The Zika virus remains a public health concern, not least because of its potential to cause birth defects and other complications. Prevention relies on mosquito control measures, education and public awareness. Ongoing research is essential to better understand the virus and develop effective prevention and treatment strategies. International cooperation is also crucial to managing epidemics and protecting vulnerable communities.[30]

COVID-19: Overview and key aspects

1. What is COVID-19?

COVID-19 is an infectious disease caused by the SARS-CoV-2 coronavirus, first identified in December 2019 in Wuhan, China. The disease rapidly led to a global pandemic, affecting millions of people and causing thousands of deaths.

2. Transmission

- **Personal transmission**: The virus is spread mainly by respiratory droplets produced when an infected person talks, coughs or sneezes.
- **Surface transmission**: It can also be spread by touching contaminated surfaces, although this is considered less frequent.
- **Aerosols**: In poorly ventilated spaces, the virus may be present in the air in the form of aerosols, increasing the risk of transmission .[31]

3. Symptoms

Symptoms of COVID-19 vary considerably, from mild to severe, and can include:

- Fever
- Cough
- Breathing difficulties
- Fatigue
- Loss of taste or smell
- Muscle pain
- Headaches

---

[30] KeesingF, Belden LK, DaszakP, Dobson A, Harvell CD, Holt RD, et al. Impacts of biodiversity on the emergence and transmission of infectious diseases. Nature. déc2010;468(7324):647-52.

[31] WoldehannaS, ZimickiS. An expanded One Health model: Integrating social science and One Health to inform study of the human-animal interface. Social Science & Medicine. March 1, 2015;129:87-95.

- Sore throat

Symptoms generally appear between 2 and 14 days after exposure to the virus.

4. Complications

- **Severe forms**: Some people may develop severe forms of the disease, including pneumonia, acute respiratory distress syndrome (ARDS) and organ failure.
- **Long COVID**: Some patients experience persistent symptoms, known as "long COVID", which can include fatigue, joint pain, cognitive impairment and respiratory problems.

5. Prevention

- **Vaccination**: Vaccines against COVID-19, such as those developed by Pfizer-BioNTech, Moderna, and Johnson & Johnson, have been deployed to reduce transmission and severe forms of the disease.
- **Sanitary measures**: Wearing masks, physical distancing, regular hand washing and the use of disinfectants are essential to reduce the spread of the virus.
- **Testing and tracing**: Regular testing and contact tracing systems have helped control epidemics.

6. Treatment

- **Supportive care**: Treatment of COVID-19 relies primarily on supportive care, including oxygen therapy and symptom management.
- **Medications**: Antivirals such as remdesivir and anti-inflammatory treatments such as corticosteroids (e.g. dexamethasone) have been used in severe cases.

7. Global Impact

- **Global pandemic**: COVID-19 has caused worldwide economic, social and health upheaval, resulting in lockdowns, school closures and disruptions to healthcare.

- **Global immunization**: Global immunization efforts have been put in place, but inequalities in access to vaccines persist between countries.

COVID-19 has transformed the global public health landscape and highlighted the importance of pandemic preparedness. Vaccination, preventive measures and case management are essential to control the spread of the virus and protect public health. The lessons learned from this pandemic will continue to inform the response to future health threats. International cooperation and solidarity are essential to overcome this global crisis and ensure a more resilient future.

M-Pox: Overview and key aspects

1. What is M-Pox?

M-Pox, formerly known as **monkeypox.** It's a viral disease caused by the orthopoxvirus. It is a member of the **Poxviridae** family. Although its name suggests an association with monkeys, the virus can infect a variety of animals and has been isolated from several species, including rodents. Although first identified in monkeys in 1958, human cases were first documented in 1970 in the Democratic Republic of Congo.

2. Transmission

- **Human transmission**: M-Pox is spread mainly by direct contact with skin lesions, body fluids or contaminated surfaces of an infected person.

3. **Animal reservoir**

- **Animal hosts**: Rodents, such as squirrels and rats, are considered the main reservoir of the virus. Monkeys may also be hosts, but they are not the main reservoir.

- **Zoonotic transmission**: Human infections generally occur through direct contact with infected animals, their blood, body fluids or skin lesions.

- **Animal reservoir**: It is also possible for the virus to be transmitted by infected animals, such as rodents.
- **Airborne transmission**: Although less common, respiratory transmission can occur in enclosed environments, mainly from respiratory droplets.

- **Global spread**: Cases of M-Pox have been reported outside Africa, notably in the USA and UK, often linked to travel or animal imports. In 2022, outbreaks in several non-endemic countries increased global concern.

5. Epidemiological implications

- **Risk profile**: The possibility of the virus spreading outside its areas of origin raises public health concerns, particularly in terms of human-to-human transmission.
- **Surveillance and prevention**: Epidemiological surveillance, awareness-raising and control measures are essential to contain epidemics and prevent transmission.

3. Symptoms

Symptoms of M-Pox in humans include:

- **Initial phase** :
  - Fever
  - Chills
  - Fatigue
  - Headaches
  - Muscle pain
- **Rash**: A few days after the onset of fever, a rash develops, often on the face, hands and genitals. Lesions evolve into papules, vesicles and pustules before forming crusts.

4. Complications

Although most infections are benign, some can lead to complications:

- **Secondary bacterial infections**: due to skin lesions.
- **Respiratory difficulties**: In rare cases, due to lung damage.
- **Mortality**: Mortality rates vary, but are higher in immunocompromised individuals.

5. Prevention

- **Case isolation**: Infected individuals must be isolated to prevent transmission.
- **Control measures**: Hygienic practices, such as hand-washing and wearing masks, are recommended to reduce the risk of spread.
- **Vaccination**: Although there is no specific vaccine for M-Pox, smallpox vaccines offer some protection due to the similarity of the viruses.

6. Treatment

- **Supportive care**: M-Pox treatment is based on supportive care, including symptom management.
- **Potential antivirals**: Drugs such as tecovirimat (TPOXX) have been used to treat severe infections.

7. Global Impact

- **Recent epidemics**: Epidemics of M-Pox have been reported in various countries, including cases outside traditionally affected regions, raising concerns about the spread of the virus.
- **Surveillance**: Health authorities closely monitor cases to control spread and respond rapidly to epidemics.

M-Pox is an emerging viral disease that requires ongoing attention in terms of surveillance and prevention. Although generally less severe than other viral diseases, its ability to spread to new regions raises public health concerns. Awareness, research and international cooperation are essential to manage this potential threat and protect vulnerable populations.

Yellow Fever Virus

Yellow Fever Virus: Overview and Key Aspects

1. What is Yellow Fever?

Yellow fever is an acute, mosquito-borne viral disease caused by the yellow fever virus, which belongs to the **Flaviviridae** family. It is endemic in certain regions of Africa and South America.

2. Transmission

- **Vector**: Mainly by mosquitoes of the genus **Aedes** (such as **Aedes aegypti**) and **Haemagogus**.
- **Human transmission**: Humans can become infected through the bites of infected mosquitoes.
- **Animal reservoir**: Non-human primates, such as monkeys, can serve as reservoirs for the virus.

3. Symptoms

Symptoms of yellow fever usually appear 3 to 6 days after infection and may include :

- **Initial phase** :
  - Fever
  - Chills
  - Headaches
  - Muscle pain
  - Nausea and vomiting
- **Regression phase**: After a few days, symptoms may improve.
- **Reinfection phase**: Approximately 15% of cases progress to a more severe form, with symptoms such as :
  - Jaundice (due to liver damage)
  - Hemorrhages (bleeding from the mouth, nose or eyes)
  - Liver and kidney failure

4. Diagnosis

Diagnosis of yellow fever is based on :

- **Travel history**: Assessment of recent travel to endemic areas.
- **Blood tests**: Detection of virus or specific antibodies by serological or PCR tests.

5. Prevention

- **Vaccination**: Vaccination is the most effective method of preventing yellow fever. The vaccine is live attenuated and provides long-lasting protection.
- **Vector control**: Reduction of mosquito populations through environmental measures and the use of repellents.
- **Education**: Raising awareness of at-risk populations about modes of transmission and protective measures.

6. Treatment

- **Supportive care**: There is no specific antiviral treatment for yellow fever. Treatment consists of supportive care, including:
  - Rehydration
  - Pain and fever management
  - Monitoring complications

7. Global Impact

- **Prevalence**: Yellow fever is endemic in tropical Africa and South America, with sporadic epidemics.
- **Mortality**: The disease can have a high mortality rate, particularly in severe cases.

Yellow fever is a preventable viral disease, thanks to vaccination and vector control measures. Awareness and prevention are essential to protect at-risk populations, particularly in endemic regions. Rapid diagnosis and appropriate care are crucial to improving patient outcomes. International cooperation is also important to monitor and control yellow fever epidemics.

Viral Meningitis Virus

Viral Meningitis Virus: Overview and Key Aspects

1. What is Viral Meningitis?

Viral meningitis is an inflammation of the meninges, the membranes enveloping the brain and spinal cord, caused by viruses. It is generally less serious than bacterial meningitis, and can often be resolved without specific treatment.

2. Pathogens

Viruses responsible for viral meningitis include :

- **Mumps virus**
- **Rubella virus**
- **Herpes viruses (HSV-1 and HSV-2)**
- **West Nile Virus**
- **Polio virus**
- **Enteroviruses (such as Coxsackie virus and echovirus)**

3. Transmission

- **Fecal-oral route**: Many enteroviruses are spread by ingestion of contaminated food or water.
- **Direct contact**: Viruses such as mumps can be transmitted through the respiratory droplets of an infected person.
- **Vector transmission**: Viruses such as West Nile virus are carried by mosquitoes.

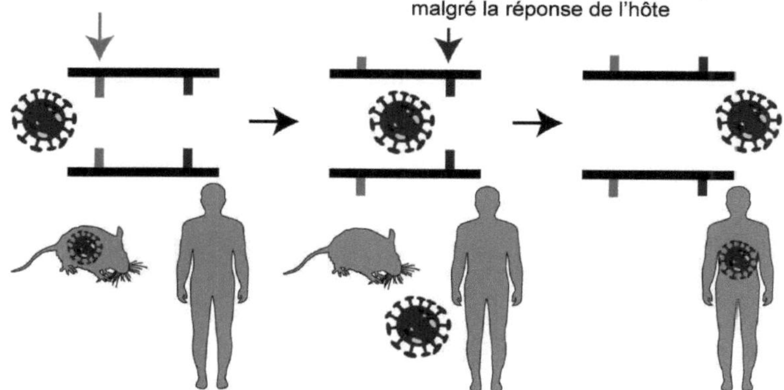

Figure 2: Encounter and compatibility filters. We have considered here an example of a virus passing from rodents to humans.

4. Symptoms

Symptoms of viral meningitis usually appear quickly and may include:

- Fever
- Severe headaches
- Stiff neck
- Photophobia (sensitivity to light)
- Nausea and vomiting
- Fatigue

5. Diagnosis

The diagnosis of viral meningitis is based on several methods:

- **Cerebrospinal fluid (CSF) analysis**: A lumbar puncture may be performed to collect CSF, which will be analyzed for signs of viral infection.

- **Blood tests**: Detection of specific antibodies or viruses in the blood.[32]

6. Prevention

- **Vaccination**: Vaccinations against mumps, rubella and other viruses can reduce the risk of viral meningitis.
- **Hygiene**: Personal hygiene practices, such as frequent hand washing, can prevent the spread of viruses.
- **Avoiding mosquito bites**: For mosquito-borne viruses, protective measures such as the use of repellents are recommended.

7. Treatment

- **Supportive care**: There is no specific antiviral treatment for viral meningitis. Treatment generally consists of symptomatic relief:
  - Analgesics for pain and fever
  - Proper hydration
- **Monitoring**: In severe cases, hospitalization may be required to monitor and treat complications.

8. Global Impact

- **Prevalence**: Viral meningitis is more common in regions where enteroviruses and other viruses are prevalent, and often accounts for a significant proportion of meningitis cases.
- **Public health**: Although generally less serious than bacterial meningitis, viral meningitis can cause complications in some individuals, particularly those with weakened immune systems.

Viral meningitis is generally a less serious infection than the bacterial form, but it does require appropriate medical attention. Vaccination and hygienic practices are essential for prevention. Early diagnosis and symptomatic treatment can help manage the disease effectively.

[32] KeesingF, Belden LK, DaszakP, Dobson A, Harvell CD, Holt RD, et al. Impacts of biodiversity on the emergence and transmission of infectious diseases. Nature. déc2010;468(7324):647-52.

Awareness-raising and education are crucial to reducing the risk of infection and protecting vulnerable populations.

Bacterial zoonoses

Leptospirosis: Overview and Key Aspects

1. What is Leptospirosis?

Leptospirosis is a bacterial infection caused by bacteria of the genus **Leptospira**. It affects a wide range of animals, including rodents, cattle, dogs and wild boar, and can be transmitted to humans. The disease occurs worldwide, but is most common in tropical and subtropical regions.

2. Transmission

- **Contact with infected animals**: Humans can become infected through direct contact with animals carrying the bacteria, especially rodents, which are the main reservoirs.
- **Contaminated water**: Leptospirosis is often spread by water contaminated with the urine of infected animals, especially in flooded areas or damp environments.
- **Soil contact**: Infection can also occur through skin or mucous membrane contact with contaminated soil or water.

3. Symptoms

Symptoms of leptospirosis vary considerably and can appear between 5 and 14 days after exposure. They include:

- **Initial phase** :
  - Fever
  - Chills
  - Headaches
  - Muscle pain
  - Nausea and vomiting

- **Advanced phase** :
  - Hemorrhagic symptoms (in severe cases)
  - Jaundice
  - Renal insufficiency
  - Meningitis
  - Weil syndrome (severe form with liver and kidney complications)

4. Diagnosis

Diagnosis of leptospirosis can be complex, as symptoms resemble those of other infections. Diagnostic methods include:

- **Serodiagnosis**: Detection of specific antibodies in the blood.
- **Culture**: Isolation of bacteria from body fluids, but this can be difficult due to the need for a specific environment.
- **Molecular tests**: PCR to detect bacterial DNA.

5. Prevention

- **Avoiding exposure**: Limit contact with potentially infected animals and avoid bathing in potentially contaminated water.
- **Rodent control**: Implement measures to reduce rodent populations in at-risk areas.
- **Education**: Raising community awareness of leptospirosis risks and prevention measures.

6. Treatment

- **Antibiotics**: Antibiotics such as penicillin or doxycycline are effective in treating leptospirosis, especially when administered early.
- **Supportive care**: In severe cases, supportive care may include hospitalization to monitor and treat complications.

7. Global Impact

- **Prevalence**: Leptospirosis is a neglected disease that is often under-diagnosed and under-reported, with thousands of cases every year worldwide.
- **Epidemics**: Epidemics can occur after floods or in animal-dense environments, endangering human populations.

Good to know: Leptospirosis is an infectious disease that can have serious consequences if not treated promptly. Prevention is based on reducing the risk of exposure and educating the population. Increased awareness and vector control efforts are essential to reduce the incidence of this disease and protect public health. Collaboration between the human, animal and environmental health sectors is crucial to better manage the risks associated with leptospirosis.

Salmonellosis: Overview and Key Aspects

1. What is Salmonellosis?

Salmonellosis is an infection caused by bacteria of the **Salmonella** genus, which are gram-negative bacteria. It is one of the main causes of foodborne infections worldwide. The two main species responsible for human infections are **Salmonella enterica** and **Salmonella bongori**.[33]

2. Transmission

- **Contaminated foods** : Transmission occurs mainly through the consumption of contaminated foods, such as :
    - Raw or undercooked meats (especially poultry and pork)
    - Raw or undercooked eggs
    - Unpasteurized dairy products
    - Contaminated fruit and vegetables

[33] Barbosa Costa G, Gilbert A, Monroe B, Blanton J, NgamNgamS, RecuencoS, et al. The influence of poverty and rabies knowledge on healthcare seeking behaviors and dog ownership, Cameroon. PLoSOne [Internet]. Jun 21, 2018 [cited 29 Apr2020];13(6). Available from: https://www.ncbi.nlm.nih.gov/pmc/articles/PMC6013156/

- **Contaminated water**: Salmonellosis can also be contracted by drinking contaminated water.
- **Contact with animals**: Reptiles, birds and some pets can carry Salmonella. Contact with these animals or their feces can also lead to infection.[34]

3. Symptoms

Symptoms of salmonellosis generally appear between 6 hours and 6 days after exposure and include :

- Diarrhea (which may be bloody)
- Fever
- Abdominal cramps
- Nausea and vomiting

The illness generally lasts from 4 to 7 days, but in some cases symptoms may persist for longer.

4. Complications

- **Dehydration**: Severe diarrhea can lead to dehydration, particularly in young children, the elderly and those with weakened immune systems.
- **Systemic infections**: In rare cases, Salmonella can enter the bloodstream and cause serious infections, such as septicemia.

5. Diagnosis

- **Laboratory tests**: The diagnosis of salmonellosis is based on laboratory tests which include :
    - Stool cultures for bacterial isolation
    - Serological tests to detect antibodies

6. Prevention

- **Food Hygiene** :

[34] CleavelandS, Sharp J, Abela-Ridder B, Allan KJ, BuzaJ, Crump JA, et al. One Health contributions towards more effective and equitable approaches to health in low-and middle-income countries. Philos Trans R Soc LondB BiolSci[Internet]. 19Jul2017 [cited 27 Apr2020];372(1725). Available from: https://www.ncbi.nlm.nih.gov/pmc/articles/PMC5468693/

- Cook meats and eggs thoroughly.
    - Avoid raw or unpasteurized foods.
    - Wash fruit and vegetables thoroughly.
- **Personal Hygiene** :
    - Wash your hands regularly, especially after handling food or animals.
- **Animal control**: Avoid contact with reptiles and ensure that pets are in good health.

7. Treatment

- **Supportive care**: Most cases of salmonellosis do not require antibiotic treatment. Treatment relies mainly on hydration to prevent dehydration.
- **Antibiotics**: In serious cases or for people at risk, antibiotics may be prescribed.

8. Global Impact

- **Epidemics**: Salmonellosis is responsible for numerous food epidemics worldwide, often linked to contaminated food products.
- **Surveillance**: Health authorities monitor epidemics to identify sources of contamination and prevent future infections.

Salmonellosis is a common but preventable foodborne infection. Awareness of food and personal hygiene is essential to reduce the risk of infection. Ongoing surveillance, prevention and education efforts are needed to protect public health and minimize the impact of Salmonella infections.

Tularemie: Overview and key aspects

1. What is Tularemie?

Tularemia is an acute bacterial infection caused by the bacterium **Francisella tularensis**. The disease can affect a variety of animals, including rodents, rabbits and deer, and can be transmitted to humans.

2. Transmission

- **Contact with infected animals**: Tularemia is generally spread by direct contact with infected animals, particularly when hunting, handling or eating game meat.
- **Insect bites**: Ticks and flies can also transmit the bacteria.[35]
- **Inhalation**: In rare cases, inhalation of contaminated aerosols can cause infection, particularly in environments where the bacterium is present in soil or agricultural activities.
- **Consumption of contaminated food or water** : Ingesting contaminated food or water can also transmit the disease.

3. Symptoms

Symptoms of tularemia may vary depending on the route of exposure and include:

- **Typical form** :
    - Fever
    - Chills
    - Fatigue
    - Headaches
    - Muscle pain
- **Localized forms** :
    - **Ulceroglandular**: formation of ulcers on the skin and swelling of lymph nodes.
    - **Oculoglandular**: Infection of the eye, causing redness, pain and discharge.
    - **Pneumonic**: Lung infection, which can cause severe respiratory symptoms.

---

35 Rahman MHAA, HaironSM, HamatRA, JamaluddinTZMT, ShafeiMN, Idris N, et al. LeptospirosisHealthIntervention Module Effecton Knowledge, Attitude, Belief, and Practice amongWetMarketWorkersin NortheasternMalaysia: An Intervention Study. Int J Environ ResPublic Health[Internet]. jul2018 [cited 2020 Jun 24];15(7). Available from: https://www.ncbi.nlm.nih.gov/pmc/articles/PMC6069487/

4. Diagnosis

The diagnosis of tularemia is based on :

- **Laboratory tests**: Culture of the bacteria from samples of blood, skin lesions or other body fluids.
- **Serological tests**: Detection of specific antibodies in the blood.

5. Prevention

- **Avoid contact with wild animals**: Limit contact with rodents and rabbits, especially when hunting or handling them.
- **Personal protection**: Use gloves and protective clothing when handling potentially infected animals.
- **Insect control**: Avoid insect bites by using repellents and wearing long clothing.

6. Treatment

- **Antibiotics**: Tularemia is usually treated with antibiotics such as streptomycin, gentamicin or doxycycline. Early treatment is essential to prevent complications.
- **Supportive care**: In severe cases, supportive care may be required.

7. Global Impact

- **Distribution**: Tularemia occurs in many parts of the world, but is most common in North America, Europe and Asia.
- **Epidemiological surveillance**: Health authorities monitor cases of tularemia to understand outbreaks and potential public health risks.

Tularemia is a potentially serious disease, but one that can be prevented with appropriate preventive measures. Awareness of the disease and its modes of transmission is essential to reduce the risk of infection. Early detection and appropriate treatment are crucial to ensure a rapid and complete recovery. Cooperation between the human and animal health sectors is also essential to control this disease.

Anthrax (Bacillus anthracis)

Anthrax (Bacillus anthracis): Overview and Key Aspects

1. What is Anthrax?

Anthrax is an acute infectious disease caused by the bacterium **Bacillus anthracis**. This bacterium forms resistant spores that can survive for long periods in the environment. Anthrax is primarily an animal disease, but it can also infect humans.

2. Transmission

Anthrax can be transmitted in several ways:

- **Direct contact**: Infection through contact with infected animals or their products (skin, hair, meat).
- **Inhalation**: Inhalation of anthrax spores, often in contaminated environments.
- **Ingestion**: Consumption of meat from infected animals that has not been properly cooked.

3. Forms of Anthrax

Anthrax takes three main forms, depending on the route of entry of the spores:

- **Cutaneous anthrax** :
  - **Transmission**: Direct contact with spores.
  - **Symptoms**: Appearance of a skin lesion (ulcer) at the site of infection, accompanied by itching, then development of a black crust. May be accompanied by fever and pain.
- **Anthrax Pulmonary** :
  - **Transmission**: Inhalation of spores.

- **Symptoms**: Initially flu-like (fever, cough, muscle aches), followed by severe breathing difficulties and shock. This is the most serious and deadly form.

- **Anthrax Gastrointestinal** :
  - **Transmission**: Ingestion of contaminated meat.
  - **Symptoms**: Nausea, vomiting, abdominal pain, diarrhea and fever. Can lead to serious complications, such as septicemia.[36]

4. Diagnosis

The diagnosis of anthrax is based on several methods:

- **Medical history**: Assessment of history of exposure to animals or animal products.
- **Laboratory tests**: Culture of the bacteria from blood samples, skin lesions or body fluids, as well as PCR tests to detect Bacillus anthracis DNA.

5. Prevention

- **Vaccination**: A vaccine is available for high-risk individuals, such as veterinary and agricultural workers.
- **Animal Control**: Surveillance and control of infected animals to prevent the spread of the disease.
- **Education**: Raising awareness of at-risk populations about modes of transmission and prevention measures.

6. Treatment

- **Antibiotics**: Antibiotics such as ciprofloxacin or penicillin are effective, especially if administered early.
- **Supportive care**: In severe cases, hospitalization may be required to treat complications, particularly in the case of pulmonary anthrax.

7. Global Impact

[36] [1] (M.) SAVEY, Commentaire de l'Agence française de sécurité sanitaire des aliments (AFSSA) In La maîtrise des maladies infectieuses, RST n° 24, Académie des sciences, 385- 387, EDP Sciences, 2006.

- **Prevalence**: Anthrax is most common in certain regions of Africa, Asia, South America and parts of Europe. It is often associated with animal husbandry.
- **Public health**: Although rare in developed countries, anthrax remains a public health concern, especially in rural areas and among people in contact with infected animals.[37]

Anthrax is a potentially fatal disease, but can be avoided through prevention, vaccination and prompt treatment. Awareness of the risks and control measures is essential to protect vulnerable populations. Ongoing surveillance and public health efforts are needed to manage this disease and reduce its impact on human and animal health.

Listeriosis

Listeriosis: Overview and Key Aspects

1. What is Listeriosis?

Listeriosis is a foodborne infection caused by the bacterium **Listeria monocytogenes**. The disease can affect healthy people, but is particularly dangerous for vulnerable groups, including pregnant women, newborns, the elderly and those with weakened immune systems.

2. Transmission

- **Consumption of contaminated food** : Listeria is often found in raw or undercooked foods, including :
  - Unpasteurized dairy products
  - Processed meats (sausages, pâtés)
  - Smoked fish
  - Contaminated fruit and vegetables
- **Cross-contamination**: The bacteria can be spread in kitchens by contaminated surfaces or utensils.

3. Symptoms

[37] [2] (V.) DEUBEL, emerging viruses In La maîtrise des maladies infectieuses, RST n° 24, Académie des sciences, 69-87, EDP Sciences, 2006.

Symptoms of listeriosis may vary depending on the severity of the infection:

- **Forme Légère** :
  - Fever
  - Headaches
  - Nausea
  - Vomiting
- **Severe form (Meningitis or Septicemia)** :
  - Flu-like symptoms
  - Stiff neck
  - Confusion or altered mental state
  - Serious complications in pregnant women, including premature delivery, abortion or stillbirth.

4. Diagnosis

The diagnosis of listeriosis is based on several methods:

- **Blood tests**: Culture of the bacteria from blood or cerebrospinal fluid samples.
- **Amniotic fluid tests**: For pregnant women, an amniotic fluid test may be carried out if infection is suspected.[38]

5. Prevention

- **Food Hygiene** :
  - Wash fruits and vegetables before eating.
  - Avoid unpasteurized dairy products.
  - Cook meat and fish thoroughly.
  - Avoid cross-contamination by cleaning surfaces and utensils.
- **Monitoring**: Food products must be monitored for the presence of Listeria, particularly in food processing establishments.

6. Treatment

[38] [4] (I.T.) EVANS, (E.G.) SMITH, (A.) BANERJEE & coll, Cluster of human tuberculosis caused by Mycobacterium bovis: Evidence for person-to-person transmission in the UK, Lancet, 2007, 369, 1270-1276.

- **Antibiotics**: Listeria infections are generally treated with antibiotics such as amoxicillin, penicillin or trimethoprim-sulfamethoxazole, particularly in severe cases.
- **Supportive care**: In cases of meningitis or septicemia, hospitalization may be required for intensive care.[39]
-

7. Global Impact

- **Prevalence**: Although less common than other foodborne infections, listeriosis can have serious consequences. It is responsible for several outbreaks, particularly in processed products.
- **Public health**: Listeriosis poses a risk to vulnerable populations, and preventive measures are crucial to reducing the incidence of this infection.

We need to be aware that listeriosis is a preventable foodborne infection, but it represents a public health challenge, particularly for at-risk groups. Awareness of food safety practices, surveillance of food products and early diagnosis are essential to prevent this disease. Prompt and appropriate treatment can reduce complications and improve patient outcomes.

Brucellosis: Overview and Key Aspects

1. What is Brucellosis?

Brucellosis is a bacterial infection caused by bacteria of the genus **Brucella**, which mainly affects farm animals such as cattle, sheep, goats and pigs. It can be transmitted to humans, often via animal products.

2. Transmission

- **Consumption of contaminated food** : Brucellosis is spread mainly through the consumption of unpasteurized dairy products and raw or undercooked meat from infected animals.

---

[39] [3] AFSSA, Rapport sur l'évaluation du risque d'apparition et de développement de maladies animales compte tenu d'un éventuel réchauffement climatique, 78 p., 2005.

- **Direct contact**: People can also become infected through direct contact with the bodily fluids of infected animals, particularly when slaughtering or handling sick animals.
- **Inhalation**: In specific work environments (such as meat processing plants), inhalation of contaminated particles can also transmit the disease.

3. Symptoms

Symptoms of brucellosis generally appear between 5 days and several months after exposure and include :

- Recurrent fever
- Chills
- Night sweats
- Fatigue
- Muscle and joint pain
- Headaches
- Weight loss

In some cases, brucellosis can lead to serious complications, such as :

- **Osteomyelitis**: Infection of the bones.
- **Endocarditis**: Infection of the heart valves.
- **Central nervous system infections**: Meningitis or brain abscess.

4. Diagnosis

Diagnosis of brucellosis is based on :

- **Laboratory tests**: Culture of the bacteria from blood or other body fluids.
- **Serological tests**: Detection of specific antibodies in the blood.

5. Prevention

- **Animal vaccination**: Vaccination of farm animals can reduce the transmission of brucellosis to humans.

- **Safe consumption**: Avoid unpasteurized dairy products and ensure that meat is thoroughly cooked.
- **Hygiene and Education**: Raising community awareness of the risks of brucellosis and appropriate hygiene practices when handling animals.

6. Treatment

- **Antibiotics**: Brucellosis is generally treated with antibiotics such as doxycycline, rifampicin or streptomycin. Prolonged treatment is often necessary to prevent relapses.
- **Supportive care**: In severe cases, medical follow-up may be required to treat complications.

7. Global Impact

- **Prevalence**: Brucellosis is considered an emerging zoonotic disease, present in many parts of the world, notably in the Mediterranean, Africa, the Middle East and Latin America.[40]
- **Epidemiological surveillance**: Health authorities monitor cases of brucellosis to understand outbreaks and prevent infections.

Brucellosis is a preventable disease that requires constant vigilance in terms of prevention and control. Awareness of transmission and prevention methods, as well as vaccination of animals, are essential to reduce the risk of infection. Early diagnosis and appropriate treatment are crucial to ensure full recovery and avoid complications. Collaboration between the animal and human health sectors is also essential to manage this zoonotic disease.

Tuberculosis: Overview and Key Aspects

1. What is tuberculosis?

Tuberculosis (TB) is a contagious bacterial infection caused by the bacterium **Mycobacterium tuberculosis**. It mainly affects the lungs, but can also affect other parts of

[40] [5] (J.) COLLINGE & (A.R.) CLARKE, A general model of prion strains and their pathogenecity, Science, 2007, 318, 930-936.

the body, such as the kidneys, spine and brain. Tuberculosis remains one of the world's leading causes of death, particularly in low- and middle-income countries.

2. Transmission

- **Airborne**: Tuberculosis is spread through the air when infected people cough, sneeze or talk, releasing droplets containing the bacteria. People nearby can inhale these droplets and contract the infection.
- **Prolonged contact**: Transmission generally requires close, prolonged contact with an infected person, making crowded environments more at risk.

3. Symptoms

Symptoms of tuberculosis can vary, but generally include:

- Persistent cough, often with bloody sputum
- Fever
- Night sweats
- Weight loss
- Fatigue
- Chest pain

Symptoms may develop slowly and be confused with other respiratory illnesses.

4. Diagnosis

The diagnosis of tuberculosis is based on several methods:

- **Skin test (Mantoux)**: Intradermal injection of a purified protein derivative (PPD) to detect an immune reaction.
- **Blood tests**: Tests such as QuantiFERON or T-SPOT to assess the immune response to tuberculosis.
- **Thoracic X-ray**: Used to detect abnormalities in the lungs.
- **Bacterial Culture**: Sputum or tissue samples are taken to culture the bacteria and confirm the diagnosis.

5. Prevention

- **Vaccination**: The BCG (Bacillus Calmette-Guérin) vaccine can offer protection against severe forms of tuberculosis in children, but its efficacy varies.
- **Infection control**: Measures such as adequate ventilation, use of masks and isolation of active cases to reduce transmission.
- **Surveillance**: Early detection of cases and follow-up of contacts are essential to control spread.

6. Treatment

- **Antibiotics**: Tuberculosis is treated with a combination of antibiotics over 6 to 9 months, usually including isoniazid, rifampicin, ethambutol and pyrazinamide.
- **Adherence to treatment**: Complete adherence to treatment is crucial to avoid the development of drug-resistant strains.

7. Global Impact

- **Prevalence**: Tuberculosis remains a global threat, with millions of cases and deaths every year. Developing countries are particularly hard hit.
- **Drug resistance** : The emergence of multidrug-resistant strains (MDR-TB) complicates treatment and calls for specific public health strategies.[41]

Tuberculosis is a preventable and treatable disease, but it continues to pose a major public health challenge. Awareness, prevention, early detection and access to treatment are essential to control TB. An integrated approach, involving collaboration between the human and animal health sectors, as well as community efforts, is crucial to reducing the impact of this disease worldwide.

[41] (N.D.) WOLFE, (C.P.) DUNAVAN & (J.) DIAMOND, origins of major human infectious diseases, Nature, 447, 279-283, 2007.

Parasitic zoonoses

Toxoplasmosis: Overview and Key Aspects

1. What is Toxoplasmosis?

Toxoplasmosis is a parasitic infection caused by the protozoan **Toxoplasma gondii**. This parasite is found worldwide and can infect a wide variety of animals, including humans. Although often asymptomatic in healthy people, toxoplasmosis can cause serious complications in immunocompromised individuals and pregnant women.[42]

2. Transmission

- **Contact with cat feces**: Cats are the parasite's definitive hosts. Transmission often occurs through contact with infected cat feces or contaminated surfaces.
- **Consumption of contaminated food** : Consumption of raw or undercooked meat, as well as unwashed fruit and vegetables, can also transmit the parasite.
- **Congenital transmission**: An infected pregnant woman can transmit the parasite to her fetus, leading to serious complications.

3. Symptoms

Most healthy people do not experience symptoms, but when symptoms do appear, they can include:

- Fever
- Fatigue
- Muscle pain
- Irritated throat
- Swollen lymph nodes

In immunocompromised individuals (such as those living with HIV/AIDS) and in newborns, toxoplasmosis can cause more severe symptoms, such as :

- Pneumonia

---

[42] [6] AFSSA - Report on H5N1 highly pathogenic avian influenza of Asian origin, 212 p., 2008 (forthcoming).

- Encephalitis
- Eye problems
- Birth defects in babies

4. Diagnosis

Diagnosis of toxoplasmosis is based on several methods:

- **Blood tests**: Detection of specific antibodies (IgG and IgM) to assess active or previous infection.
- **Imaging**: In severe cases, imaging tests (such as CT or MRI scans) may be used to detect brain lesions.

5. Prevention

- **Hygiene** :
  - Wash hands after handling cat feces or raw food.
  - Avoid changing cat litter during pregnancy, or wear gloves.
- **Cooking food**: Cook meat thoroughly and wash fruit and vegetables before eating.
- **Avoiding stray cats**: Reduce the risk of exposure by avoiding unidentified or stray cats.

6. Treatment

- **Antiparasitic agents**: Treatment of toxoplasmosis may include drugs such as pyrimethamine and sulfadiazine, often combined with folic acid to reduce side effects.
- **Follow-up**: Immunocompromised people may need prophylactic treatment to avoid infection.

7. Global Impact

- **Prevalence**: Toxoplasmosis is a common infection worldwide, with high prevalence in many populations.
- **Public health**: Although often asymptomatic, toxoplasmosis can have a significant impact on pregnant women and immunocompromised people, making it a public health concern.

Toxoplasmosis is a widespread but often overlooked infection. Awareness of modes of transmission and preventive measures is essential to reduce the risk of infection, particularly in vulnerable populations. Early diagnosis and appropriate treatment are crucial to managing this infection and preventing serious complications. A proactive approach involving education and prevention can help reduce the impact of toxoplasmosis in the community.

Chagas disease: Overview and key aspects

1. What is Chagas disease?

Chagas disease is a parasitic infection caused by the protozoan **Trypanosoma cruzi**. It was first described by the Brazilian physician Carlos Chagas in 1909. The disease is mainly endemic in Latin America, but is also a growing risk in other regions due to migration.

2. Transmission

- **Insect bites**: The disease is mainly transmitted by triatomine insects, also known as "bedbugs" or "triatomine bugs". These insects become infected by feeding on the blood of infected animals or humans, and transmit the parasite through their excrement.
- **Blood transmission**: It can also be spread by blood transfusion, organ transplantation or from mother to child during pregnancy.
- **Consumption of contaminated food**: In some cases, contamination of food by the excrement of infected insects can also be a route of transmission.

3. Symptoms

Chagas disease develops in two phases:

- **Acute phase**: This phase may last a few weeks or months and may be asymptomatic. When symptoms do appear, they include :
  - Fever
  - Fatigue
  - Muscle pain
  - Swelling at the bite site (chagoma)
  - Skin rash

- **Chronic phase**: This can occur years after the initial infection. Around 20-30% of people develop complications, such as :
  - Heart problems (cardiomyopathy)
  - Digestive disorders (dilatation of the oesophagus or colon)
  - Neurological problems

4. Diagnosis

The diagnosis of Chagas disease is based on several methods:

- **Blood tests**: Detection of the parasite or specific antibodies in the blood.
- **Clinical examination**: Assessment of symptoms and exposure history.

5. Prevention

- **Insect control**: Measures to reduce the triatomine insect population, including improved housing conditions and the use of insecticides.
- **Education**: Raising awareness of at-risk populations about modes of transmission and preventive measures.
- **Screening**: Screening of blood donors and pregnant women to reduce transmission.

6. Treatment

- **Antiparasitic agents**: drugs such as benznidazole and nifurtimox are used to treat infection, particularly in the acute phase.
- **Symptomatic care**: In the chronic phase, treatment focuses on managing symptoms and complications, including heart problems.

7. Global Impact

- **Prevalence**: Chagas disease affects millions of people, mainly in Latin America, but cases are reported in other regions, including the United States and Europe, due to migration.
- **Burden of disease**: The disease represents a significant public health burden, particularly in at-risk communities.

Chagas disease is a preventable and treatable parasitic infection, but it continues to pose a public health challenge in many regions. Awareness of modes of transmission, prevention and early detection are essential in the fight against this disease. An integrated approach, involving community efforts and collaboration between the human and animal health sectors, is crucial to reducing the impact of Chagas disease and protecting vulnerable populations.

Echinococcosis: Overview and Key Aspects

1. What is Echinococcosis?

Echinococcosis is a parasitic infection caused by tapeworms of the genus **Echinococcus**. The two main species responsible for the disease in humans are **Echinococcus granulosus** and **Echinococcus multilocularis**. This infection can cause cysts to form in various organs, notably the liver and lungs.

2. Transmission

- **Contact with infected animals**: Echinococcosis is transmitted mainly through contact with infected animals, particularly dogs and other carnivores. Animals excrete the parasite's eggs in their feces.
- **Ingestion of eggs**: Humans can become infected by ingesting eggs present in contaminated food, water or surfaces, often by handling animals or their excrement.
- **Environmental transmission**: Eggs can survive in the environment, particularly in soil or on plants, increasing the risk of infection.

3. Symptoms

The symptoms of echinococcosis depend on the location and size of the cysts. Forms of the disease include:

- **Cystic echinococcosis (E. granulosus)** :
  - Cysts usually asymptomatic for years.
  - Symptoms may include abdominal pain, nausea, and symptoms due to organ compression.
- **Alveolar echinococcosis (E. multilocularis)** :

- More aggressive form, often mistaken for liver cancer.
- Symptoms include abdominal pain, weight loss, jaundice, and ascites (accumulation of fluid in the abdomen).

4. Diagnosis

Diagnosis of echinococcosis is based on several methods:

- **Imaging**: Ultrasound, computed tomography (CT) or magnetic resonance imaging (MRI) to detect cysts in organs.
- **Blood tests**: Detection of specific antibodies against the parasite.
- **Biopsy**: In some cases, a biopsy may be required to confirm the diagnosis.

5. Prevention

- **Education and awareness**: Inform at-risk populations about modes of transmission and prevention measures.
- **Hygiene**: Wash hands after handling animals and avoid consumption of potentially contaminated food or water.[43]
- **Animal control**: Keep dogs out of areas where farm animals are kept, and treat pets for parasitic infections.

6. Treatment

- **Surgery**: In many cases, surgical removal of cysts is the treatment of choice.
- **Antiparasitic drugs**: Drugs such as albendazole or mebendazole can be used, but they do not replace surgery for established cysts.

7. Global Impact

- **Prevalence**: Echinococcosis is more prevalent in rural and livestock areas, particularly in South America, Europe, Asia and Africa.

[43] (N.D.) WOLFE, (C.P.) DUNAVAN & (J.) DIAMOND, origins of major human infectious diseases, Nature, 447, 279-283, 2007.

- **Burden of disease**: This is a public health problem, due to the complications it can cause and its economic impact on healthcare systems.

Echinococcosis is a preventable parasitic infection, but it requires ongoing vigilance in terms of prevention and control. Awareness of the risk of infection, hygiene measures and appropriate treatment of pets are essential to reduce the incidence of this disease. Early diagnosis and appropriate treatment are crucial to minimizing complications and improving patient outcomes. An integrated approach involving public health, animal husbandry and community education is essential to combat echinococcosis.

Cysticercosis

Cysticercosis: Overview and Key Aspects

1. What is cysticercosis?

Cysticercosis is a parasitic infection caused by the larvae of the tapeworm *Taenia solium*, also known as pork tapeworm. This disease occurs when humans ingest eggs of this parasite, often through contaminated food or water.

2. Transmission

- **Egg ingestion**: Transmission occurs mainly through ingestion *of Taenia solium* eggs, which may be found in food or water contaminated with human excrement.
- **Contact with infected pigs**: Pigs can harbor the adult tapeworm, and their consumption of undercooked meat can also be a source of infection.

3. Life cycle

1. **Ingestion of eggs**: When a human ingests eggs, they develop into larvae and enter the bloodstream.
2. **Cyst formation**: Larvae migrate to various tissues, including the brain, eyes and muscles, where they form cysts.
3. **Cysts**: These cysts can remain asymptomatic for years, but they can also cause severe symptoms.

4. Symptoms

The symptoms of cysticercosis depend on the location of the cysts. The most common forms include :

- **Neurocysticercosis** (cysts in the brain) :
  - Convulsions
  - Headaches
  - Neurological symptoms (confusion, balance disorders, etc.)
- **Cysts in other tissues** :
  - Muscle pain
  - Localized swelling

5. Diagnosis

Diagnosis of cysticercosis is based on several methods:

- **Medical Imaging** :
  - **MRI or CT**: To visualize cysts in the brain or other organs.
- **Blood tests**: Search for specific antibodies against *Taenia solium.*
- **Medical history**: Assessment of history of consumption of undercooked pork or potential exposure to human excrement.

6. Prevention

- **Hygiene**: rigorous hygiene practices, including hand washing and proper management of human excrement.
- **Food safety**: fully cook pork and avoid consumption of uncooked products.
- **Education**: Raising awareness of at-risk populations about modes of transmission and preventive measures.

7. Treatment

- **Antiparasitic drugs**: Drugs such as albendazole or praziquantel can be used to treat infections.
- **Treatment of symptoms**: In cases of neurocysticercosis, anti-epileptic drugs may be needed to control convulsions.
- **Surgical intervention**: In some cases, surgery may be required to remove cysts, especially if they are causing severe symptoms.

8. Global Impact

- **Prevalence**: Cysticercosis is common in regions where hygiene is poor and pork consumption is high, notably in Latin America, Africa and Asia.
- **Public health**: Neurocysticercosis is a major public health problem, particularly because of the neurological complications associated with it.

Cysticercosis is a preventable parasitic infection, but it remains a public health challenge in many parts of the world. Prevention relies on rigorous hygiene practices, adequate food safety and education of at-risk populations. Early diagnosis and appropriate treatment are crucial to minimizing complications and improving patient outcomes.

Leishmaniasis: Overview and Key Aspects

1. What is Leishmaniasis?

Leishmaniasis is a parasitic disease caused by protozoa of the genus *Leishmania*. It is transmitted to humans through the bite of sandflies, mosquito-like insects. Leishmaniasis has several clinical forms, the most common of which are cutaneous and visceral leishmaniasis.

2. Transmission

- **Vector**: Transmission is mainly via the bite of infected sandflies.
- **Animal reservoirs**: Disease reservoirs include a variety of animals, such as dogs, rodents and other mammals.

3. Forms of Leishmaniasis

a. Cutaneous leishmaniasis

- **Symptoms** :
  - Skin lesions, often in the form of ulcers.
  - Skin rashes that may be painful.
  - May cause scarring.

b. Visceral leishmaniasis (Kala-azar)

- **Symptoms** :
  - Prolonged fever.
  - Significant weight loss.
  - Anemia.
  - Splenomegaly (enlarged spleen) and hepatomegaly (enlarged liver).
  - Can be fatal if left untreated.

4. Diagnosis

Diagnosis of leishmaniasis is based on several methods:

- **Clinical examination**: Assessment of symptoms and history of sandfly bites.

- **Laboratory tests** :
  - **Culture**: cultivation of the parasite from skin lesions or blood samples.
  - **Biopsy**: Biopsy of skin lesions or internal organs to identify the parasite.
  - **Blood tests**: Serological tests to detect specific antibodies.

5. Prevention

- **Vector control**: Measures to reduce the sandfly population, such as the use of repellents, improved housing and mosquito nets.
- **Education**: Raising awareness of at-risk populations about modes of transmission and preventive measures.
- **Animal protection**: Monitoring and treatment of domestic animals to reduce the risk of transmission.[44]

6. Treatment

- **Antiparasitic drugs** :
  - **Antimonials** (such as sodium stibogluconate) are often used to treat visceral and cutaneous leishmaniasis.

---

[44] (N.D.) WOLFE, (C.P.) DUNAVAN & (J.) DIAMOND, origins of major human infectious diseases, Nature, 447, 279-283, 2007.

- **Amphotericin B**: Used in severe cases, notably visceral leishmaniasis.
- **Miltefosine**: An oral medication for the treatment of certain forms of leishmaniasis.

- **Supportive care**: In severe cases, hospitalization may be required for intensive monitoring and treatment.

7. Global Impact

- **Prevalence**: Leishmaniasis is endemic in many parts of the world, notably Latin America, Africa, Asia and Southern Europe.
- **Public health**: It represents a major public health problem, particularly in rural areas and among vulnerable populations.

Worth knowing: Leishmaniasis is a preventable and treatable parasitic disease, but it requires special attention in terms of prevention, awareness and treatment. International cooperation and public health efforts are essential to control the spread of this disease and protect populations at risk. Early diagnosis and appropriate treatment are crucial to improving patient outcomes and reducing the morbidity associated with this infection.[45]

Giardiosis: Overview and Key Aspects

1. What is Giardiosis?

Giardiosis is an intestinal infection caused by the protozoan *Giardia lamblia* (or *Giardia intestinalis*). The disease is one of the most common causes of diarrhoea worldwide, affecting both children and adults.[46]

---

[45] Canadian Food Inspection Agency. (2003b). Rapport annuel, Questionnaire FAO/ OIE/ OMS - 2003, Canada, Report submitted to the Office International des Épizooties. Available February 22, 2006 at www.inspection.gc.ca/francais/anima/surv/ 2003oief. shtml

[46] Canadian Food Inspection Agency. (2005). Hantavirus pulmonary syndrome. Accessed October 18, 2005 at www.inspection.gc.ca/francais/anima/heasan/disemala/ hanta/hantafsf.shtml

2. Transmission

- **Fecal-oral route**: Giardiosis is transmitted mainly by ingestion of *Giardia* cysts, present in :
    - Contaminated water (springs, rivers or untreated water).
    - Contaminated food.
    - Contact with contaminated surfaces or objects.
- **Person-to-person contact**: Can also occur in collective environments, such as day-care centers or institutions.

3. Symptoms

Symptoms of giardiosis vary from person to person, and may appear 1 to 3 weeks after infection. They include:

- Diarrhea (may be watery and odorous)
- Abdominal pain and cramps
- Bloating
- Nausea
- Fatigue
- Weight loss
- Nutrient malabsorption

Some people may be asymptomatic, but they can still transmit the infection.

4. Diagnosis

The diagnosis of giardiosis is based on several methods:

- **Stool analysis**: Identification of *Giardia* cysts or trophozoites in stool samples.
- **Laboratory tests**: Specific tests can be carried out, such as PCR (polymerase chain reaction) to detect the parasite's DNA.

5. Prevention

- **Hygiene** :
    - Wash your hands regularly, especially before eating and after using the toilet.
    - Avoid consuming untreated water or ice made from potentially contaminated water.
- **Food safety** :

- Wash fruit and vegetables thoroughly before eating.
- Cook food at appropriate temperatures to kill parasites.

- **Education**: Raising awareness of at-risk populations about modes of transmission and preventive measures.

6. Treatment

- **Antiparasitic drugs** :
  - **Metronidazole**, **Tinidazole** and **Nitazoxanide** are commonly prescribed to treat giardiosis.
- **Hydration**: Maintaining good hydration is essential, especially in cases of severe diarrhea.

7. Global Impact

- **Prevalence**: Giardiosis is particularly common in areas where hygiene is poor and access to drinking water is limited. It is also common in camping areas and rural environments.
- **Public health**: Although generally not fatal, giardiosis can lead to complications, particularly in immunocompromised individuals and young children.

Giardiosis is a preventable and treatable intestinal infection, but it requires special attention in terms of prevention, awareness and treatment. Maintaining good hygiene practices and food safety are essential to reduce the risk of transmission. Early diagnosis and appropriate treatment can relieve symptoms and improve patient outcomes.

Balanocephalosis: Overview and Key Aspects

1. What is Balanocephalosis?

Balanocephalosis, also known as **bilanocephalosis**, is a parasitic infection caused by flatworms of the *Echinococcus* genus, notably *Echinococcus granulosus* and *Echinococcus multilocularis*. The disease is characterized by the formation of cysts in various organs, mainly the liver and lungs.[47]

2. Transmission

- **Life cycle**: Humans act as intermediate hosts. Transmission occurs mainly through ingestion *of Echinococcus* eggs, which can be found in :
  - Feces from dogs or other infected animals (main reservoirs).
  - Contaminated food or water.

3. Types of Echinococcosis

There are two main types of echinococcosis:

a. Cystic echinococcosis (Echinococcus granulosus)

- **Cysts** : Form of hydatid cysts in internal organs.
- **Symptoms**: Often asymptomatic at first; symptoms may appear when cysts become enlarged, causing abdominal pain, jaundice, or respiratory symptoms depending on their location.

b. Alveolar echinococcosis (Echinococcus multilocularis)

- **Cysts**: Form more invasive, tumor-like cysts that can spread locally.
- **Symptoms**: May include abdominal pain, weight loss, and liver symptoms, similar to those of a malignant tumor.

4. Diagnosis

The diagnosis of balanocephalosis is based on several methods:

- **Medical Imaging** :
  - **Ultrasound**, CT (computed tomography) or **MRI** to visualize cysts in organs.
- **Blood tests**: Search for specific antibodies against *Echinococcus*.

---

[47] Canadian Food Inspection Agency. (2003a). Rabies. Accessed November 2, 2005 at www.inspection.gc.ca/ english/anima/heasan/disemala/rabrag/rabragfsf.shtml

- **Medical history**: Assessment of history of exposure to infected animals or contaminated environments.

5. Prevention

- **Hygiene**: Wash hands after handling animals or animal excrement.
- **Education**: Raising awareness among at-risk populations, especially dog breeders, of the modes of transmission.
- **Animal Control**: Regular deworming of dogs and other pets.

6. Treatment

- **Antiparasitic drugs** :
  - **Albendazole** or **Mebendazole** to treat the infection.
- **Surgery**: In many cases, surgery may be required to remove cysts, especially if complications arise.

7. Global Impact

- **Prevalence**: Balanocephalosis is most common in rural areas and among populations in close contact with infected animals, particularly in parts of Europe, Asia and Africa.
- **Public health**: Although often preventable, it can have serious consequences, especially if not diagnosed and treated promptly.[48]

Balanocephalosis is a serious but preventable parasitic infection, requiring awareness, education and prevention efforts. Maintaining good hygiene practices and early diagnosis are essential to reduce the risk of infection and improve patient outcomes. A proactive approach to managing animal populations and contaminated environments is crucial to controlling this disease.

Filariasis: Overview and Key Aspects

1. What is Filariasis?

[48] Public Health Agency of Canada (2006). Notifiable diseases online - Rabies. Accessed February 22, 2006 at http://dsol-smed.phac aspc.gc.ca/dsol-smed/ ndis/disease2/ rabi_e.html

Filariasis is a parasitic infection caused by roundworms (nematodes) belonging to the genera *Wuchereria*, *Brugia* and others. These parasites are transmitted to humans through the bites of insect vectors, mainly mosquitoes.[49]

2. Types of Filariasis

There are several forms of filariasis, the most common being :

a. Lymphatic Filariasis

- **Pathogens**: *Wuchereria bancrofti*, *Brugia malayi.*
- **Transmission**: Bites of infected mosquitoes.
- **Symptoms** :
  - Swelling of limbs (elephantiasis).
  - Pain in lymph nodes.
  - Fever.
  - Tissue inflammation.

b. Onchocerciasis (river blindness)

- **Pathogen**: *Onchocerca volvulus.*
- **Transmission**: Black fly bites (Simulium).
- **Symptoms** :
  - Intense itching.
  - Skin lesions.
  - Blindness due to eye infections.

c. Loasis (Loa loa filariasis)

- **Pathogen**: *Loa loa.*
- **Transmission**: Bites of kite flies (Chrysops).
- **Symptoms** :
  - Visible migration of worms under the skin.
  - Eye inflammation (conjunctivitis) and joint pain.

3. Diagnosis

[49] Public Health Agency of Canada (2005a). Disease Information - Malaria. Accessed October 20, 2005 at www. phac-aspc.gc.ca/tmp-pmv/info/pal_mal_e.html

The diagnosis of filariasis is based on several methods:

- **Blood analysis**: Detection of microfilaria in blood, usually by thick drop or concentration technique.
- **Medical imaging**: Ultrasound to visualize adult worms, particularly in the case of lymphatic filariasis.
- **Laboratory tests**: Tissue biopsies or skin samples for worm identification.

4. Prevention

- **Vector control**: Reduction of the mosquito and fly population through insecticides and sanitation measures.
- **Personal protection**: Use mosquito nets, repellents and long clothing to avoid bites.
- **Education**: Raising awareness of at-risk populations about modes of transmission and preventive measures.

5. Treatment

- **Antiparasitic drugs** :
  - **Diethylcarbamazine (DEC)**: Used to treat lymphatic filariasis.
  - **Ivermectin**: Used for onchocerciasis and sometimes for other forms.
  - **Albendazole**: Can be used in combination with other treatments.
- **Supportive care**: In cases of elephantiasis, treatment to reduce swelling and improve quality of life may be required.

6. Global Impact

- **Prevalence**: Filariasis is endemic in many tropical and subtropical regions, affecting millions of people worldwide, particularly in Africa, Asia and South America.
- **Public health**: Although not often fatal, filariasis can cause significant disability, affecting the quality of life and productivity of those infected.

7. Conclusion

Filariasis is a preventable and treatable parasitic disease, but it requires special attention in terms of prevention, education and treatment. Vector control, good hygiene practices and increased awareness are essential to reduce the risk of infection. Early diagnosis and appropriate treatment are crucial to improving patient outcomes and minimizing the complications associated with this disease.[50]

Schistosomiasis: Overview and Key Aspects

1. What is Schistosomiasis?

Schistosomiasis, also known as bilharzia, is a parasitic infection caused by flatworms of the genus *Schistosoma*. The disease is endemic in many tropical and subtropical regions, affecting millions of people worldwide.

2. Transmission

- **Life cycle**: Transmission occurs mainly through contact with freshwater contaminated by schistosome larvae (cercariae), which penetrate the skin of people who swim or bathe in infected water.
- **Intermediate hosts**: Freshwater snails act as intermediate hosts, housing larvae before they are released into the water.

3. Types of Schistosomiasis

There are several species of schistosomes, but the most common are :

a. Schistosoma mansoni

- **Location**: Africa, South America, Caribbean.
- **Symptoms** :
  - Diarrhea, abdominal pain and hemorrhoids.
  - May cause liver complications.

b. Schistosoma haematobium

- **Location**: Africa, Middle East.

[50] Public Health Agency of Canada (2005b). News briefs for infectious diseases. Available November 11, 2005 at www.phac-aspc.gc.ca/bid bmi/dsddsm/ nb-ab/index_e. html

- **Symptoms** :
  - Blood in the urine (hematuria).
  - Pain during urination and urinary tract infections.

c. Schistosoma japonicum

- **Location**: East Asia (China, Philippines).
- **Symptoms** :
  - Similar to *S. mansoni*, but can also cause gastrointestinal complications.

4. Symptoms

Symptoms of schistosomiasis may vary depending on the stage of infection:

- **Acute phase** (4 to 6 weeks after exposure) :
  - Allergic reaction: itching, rash, fever and muscle pain.
- **Chronic phase** :
  - Symptoms related to the organ affected (liver, intestines, bladder).
  - Abdominal pain, diarrhea, blood in stools or urine, and liver complications.

5. Diagnosis

The diagnosis of schistosomiasis is based on several methods:

- **Stool or urine analysis**: Detection of schistosome eggs in samples.
- **Blood tests**: Search for specific antibodies or antigens.
- **Medical imaging**: Ultrasound or CT scan to assess organ damage.

6. Prevention

- **Avoid contact with contaminated water**: Avoid swimming or bathing in fresh water suspected of being contaminated.
- **Sanitation** : Improving sanitation facilities to reduce contamination.
- **Education**: Raising awareness of risks and prevention measures.

7. Treatment

- **Antiparasitic drugs** :
  - **Praziquantel**: The main treatment for all forms of schistosomiasis, effective in killing adult worms.
- **Supportive care**: Treatment of complications related to affected organs and symptom management.

8. Global Impact

- **Prevalence**: Schistosomiasis is endemic in around 78 countries, affecting over 200 million people, mainly in Africa, Asia and South America.[51]
- **Public health**: It is considered a major health problem, contributing to morbidity and impacting on economic development in affected regions.

Schistosomiasis is a preventable and treatable parasitic disease, but it requires special attention in terms of prevention, education and treatment. Vector control, improved health infrastructures and increased awareness are essential to reduce the risk of infection. Early diagnosis and appropriate treatment are crucial to minimizing complications and improving patient outcomes.

Anisakidosis: Overview and Key Aspects

1. What is Anisakidosis?

Anisakidosis is a parasitic infection caused by larvae of nematode worms of the genus *Anisakis*, found mainly in fish and seafood. This disease can cause gastrointestinal symptoms in humans after eating raw or undercooked fish.

2. Transmission

- **Consumption of contaminated fish** : Infection occurs mainly through ingestion of *Anisakis* larvae present in :
  - Raw or undercooked fish (such as herring, mackerel and salmon).

---

[51] Public Health Agency of Canada (2005d). Notifiable diseases online. Available November 3, 2005 at http://dsol-smed.phac-aspc.gc.ca/dsol smed/ndis/ list_f. html#tab2<

- Seafood, especially squid.

3. Symptoms

Symptoms of anisakidosis may appear a few hours after ingesting infected larvae:

- **Gastrointestinal symptoms** :
  - Acute abdominal pain.
  - Nausea and vomiting.
  - Diarrhea.
  - Feeling of discomfort.
- **Allergic reactions**: In some cases, the infection may cause allergic reactions, such as itching or rashes.

4. Diagnosis

Diagnosis of anisakidosis is based on several methods:

- **Food history**: Assessment of history of consumption of raw or undercooked fish.
- **Medical imaging**: Ultrasound, CT or endoscopy to visualize larvae in the digestive tract.
- **Blood tests**: Testing for specific antibodies to *Anisakis*.

5. Prevention

- **Cooking instructions**: Cook fish at a temperature of at least 63°C (145°F) to kill larvae.
- **Freezing**: Freeze fish at -20°C (-4°F) for at least 7 days before eating raw, to kill larvae.
- **Education**: Raising consumer awareness of the risks involved in eating raw fish.

6. Treatment

- **Symptomatic**: Treatment is generally symptomatic, including analgesics to relieve abdominal pain.
- **Medical intervention**: In severe cases, endoscopy may be required to remove the larvae.

7. Global Impact

- **Prevalence**: Anisakidosis is more prevalent in regions where raw fish consumption is common, such as Japan, Europe and North America.
- **Public health**: Although anasakidosis is generally benign, it can lead to complications in rare cases, requiring medical attention.

8. Conclusion

Anisakidosis is a parasitic infection that can be prevented by proper food safety practices. Proper cooking of fish and consumer awareness are essential to prevent this disease. Prompt diagnosis and appropriate treatment can relieve symptoms and avoid complications.

Fungal zoonoses

Histoplasmosis: Overview and Key Aspects

1. What is Histoplasmosis?

Histoplasmosis is a fungal infection caused by the fungus **Histoplasma capsulatum**. This fungus is found mainly in soil, often in association with bird or bat droppings. The infection is common in certain regions of the United States and other parts of the world.

2. Transmission

- **Inhalation of fungal spores**: Transmission occurs mainly through inhalation of microscopic spores (conidia) present in the air, often when the soil is disturbed (e.g. during construction or gardening work).
- **Contaminated environment**: Areas where birds or bats live are at risk, as debris from these animals can carry the fungus.

3. Symptoms

Symptoms of histoplasmosis can vary considerably, from asymptomatic forms to severe infections:

- **Acute form** :
  - Fever

- Dry cough
- Chest pain
- Fatigue
- Chills

- **Chronic form**: May resemble tuberculosis, with symptoms such as :
  - Persistent cough
  - Expectoration of mucus or blood
  - Weight loss
  - Night sweats
- **Disseminated form**: Occurs mainly in immunocompromised individuals and may affect several organs. Symptoms may include:
  - High fever
  - Anemia
  - Severe respiratory problems

4. Diagnosis

The diagnosis of histoplasmosis is based on several methods:

- **Blood tests**: Detection of specific antibodies or fungal antigens in blood or urine.
- **Imaging**: X-ray or computed tomography (CT) to assess the lungs.
- **Culture**: Cultivation of the fungus from blood, mucus or tissue samples.

5. Prevention

- **Avoid Risk Areas**: Limit exposure to environments where the fungus is likely to be present, such as construction zones or caves.
- **Personal protection**: Use masks and protective clothing when working in potentially contaminated areas.
- **Education**: Raising awareness of at-risk populations about modes of transmission and preventive measures.

6. Treatment

- **Antifungals**: Treatment of acute or chronic histoplasmosis may include antifungal drugs such as itraconazole or voriconazole. In severe cases, drugs such as amphotericin B may be necessary.

- **Supportive care**: In severe cases, hospitalization may be required to monitor and manage complications.

7. Global Impact

- **Prevalence**: Histoplasmosis is most common in regions of the United States such as Ohio and Mississippi, as well as in parts of Latin America and Asia.
- **Public health**: Although often benign, histoplasmosis can have serious consequences in immunocompromised individuals, making it a public health concern.

8. Conclusion

Histoplasmosis is a preventable and treatable fungal infection, but it requires awareness and appropriate preventive measures. Knowledge of the risks and environments at risk, as well as the use of adequate protection, are essential to reduce the incidence of this disease. Early diagnosis and appropriate treatment are crucial to improving outcomes for patients, particularly those at high risk. An integrated approach involving education and public health is essential to effectively combat histoplasmosis.

Cryptococcosis: Overview and Key Aspects

1. What is Cryptococcosis?

Cryptococcosis is a fungal infection caused by the fungus **Cryptococcus neoformans** and, less frequently, **Cryptococcus gattii**. The disease is mainly associated with immunocompromised individuals, notably those living with HIV/AIDS, but can also affect healthy individuals.

2. Transmission

- **Inhalation of spores**: Transmission occurs mainly through inhalation of fungal spores present in the environment, often in places where pigeon or other bird droppings are found.

- **Environmental factors**: The fungus is widely present in soil and decomposing organic matter.

3. Symptoms

Symptoms of cryptococcosis can vary considerably depending on the location of the infection:

- **Pulmonary cryptococcosis** :
  - Persistent cough
  - Fever
  - Chest pain
  - Shortness of breath
- **Cryptococcal meningitis**: This is the most serious form, which can lead to major complications:
  - Severe headaches
  - Stiff neck
  - Fever
  - Confusion or altered mental state
  - Photophobia (sensitivity to light)
- **Skin infection**: Skin lesions may appear, but are less frequent.

4. Diagnosis

The diagnosis of cryptococcosis is based on several methods:

- **Blood tests**: Detection of specific antigens in blood or cerebrospinal fluid (CSF).
- **Culture**: Cultivation of the fungus from lung, CSF or other samples.
- **Imaging**: X-ray or computed tomography (CT) to assess the lungs and detect any lesions.

5. Prevention

- **Exposure control**: Avoid high-risk environments, especially those where bird droppings are present.
- **Monitoring People at Risk**: Immunocompromised people should be closely monitored for signs of infection.

- **Preventive treatment**: People living with HIV/AIDS can benefit from prophylactic treatment to prevent infection.[52]

6. Treatment

- **Antifungals**: Treatment of cryptococcosis generally involves antifungal drugs, such as :
  - **Amphotericin B**: Used for severe infections.
  - **Flucytosine**: often administered in association with amphotericin.
  - **Fluconazole**: Used for maintenance treatment after initial infection.
- **Supportive care**: In severe cases, hospitalization may be required to monitor and treat complications.

7. Global Impact

- **Prevalence**: Cryptococcosis is a common fungal infection, particularly among immunocompromised people worldwide.
- **Public health**: It represents a public health problem, especially in developing countries where HIV/AIDS is more widespread.

8. Conclusion

Cryptococcosis is a preventable and treatable fungal infection, but it requires increased awareness and preventive measures, particularly for at-risk populations.[53] Early diagnosis and appropriate treatment are crucial to improving patient outcomes. An integrated approach involving public health, education and research is essential to combat this disease and reduce its impact on global health.

---

[52] Bouden M., Moulin, B., Gosselin, P., Back, C., Doyon, B., Gingras, D. & Lebel, G. (2005). Geo-simulation of West Nile virus infection as a function of climate: a public health risk management tool. C-CIARN Conference 2005. Adapting to Climate Change in Canada 2005: Understanding the Risks and Building Capacity. Montreal. May 4-7, 2005.

[53] Binder S., A M Levitt, and J M Hughes (1999). Preventing emerging infectious diseases as we enter the 21st century: CDC's strategy. Public Health Rep. Mar-Apr; 114(2): 130- 134.

Candidiasis

Candidiasis: Overview and Key Aspects

1. What is Candidiasis?

Candidiasis is a fungal infection caused by fungi of the *Candida* genus, in particular *Candida albicans*. Although *Candida* is a normal part of the human microbial flora, excessive overgrowth can lead to infection.

2. Types of Candidiasis

Candidiasis can take many forms, including :

a. Oral candidiasis (thrush)

- **Symptoms**: White lesions in the mouth, pain and difficulty swallowing.
- **At-risk population**: infants, immunocompromised people and those with dentures.

b. Vaginal candidiasis

- **Symptoms**: Itching, thick, white vaginal discharge, pain during intercourse.
- **Risk factors**: use of antibiotics, pregnancy, diabetes and weakened immune systems.

c. Systemic candidiasis

- **Symptoms**: Serious infection that can affect several organs, leading to fever, chills and deterioration of general condition.
- **At-risk population**: patients in hospital, with intravenous devices or immunocompromised.

3. Transmission

- **Endogenous**: Candidiasis is often caused by an overgrowth *of Candida* already present in the body.
- **Environment**: In some cases, infection can be caused by exposure to damp or contaminated environments.

4. Diagnosis

The diagnosis of candidiasis is based on several methods:

- **Clinical examination**: Assessment of symptoms and medical history.
- **Laboratory tests** :
  - Tissue or secretion samples for *Candida* culture and identification.
  - Blood tests to diagnose systemic infections.

5. Prevention

- **Hygiene**: Maintain good body and oral hygiene, in particular by keeping the mouth and genital area dry.
- **Diet**: Reduce consumption of sugars and processed foods, which can promote *Candida* overgrowth.
- **Avoid unnecessary antibiotics**: Limit the use of antibiotics, which can unbalance microbial flora.

6. Treatment

- **Antifungals** :
  - **Topical**: Antifungal creams or ointments for cutaneous and vaginal candidiasis.
  - **Systemic**: Oral or intravenous medications (such as fluconazole) for more serious or systemic infections.
- **Supportive care**: management of symptoms and risk factors, such as glycemic control for diabetics.

7. Global Impact

- **Prevalence**: Candidiasis is common and can affect anyone, but is more common in immunocompromised people.
- **Public health**: Although generally treatable, systemic infections can be serious and require urgent medical attention.

8. Conclusion

Candidiasis is a preventable and treatable fungal infection. Awareness of risk factors, hygiene, and the importance of appropriate treatment is essential to prevent and manage this infection. Early diagnosis and appropriate treatment are crucial to improving patient outcomes and minimizing the complications associated with candidiasis.

Aspergillosis: Overview and Key Aspects

1. What is Aspergillosis?

Aspergillosis is a fungal infection caused by fungi of the genus *Aspergillus*. It can affect various organs, mainly the lungs, and is of particular concern in immunocompromised individuals.

2. Types of Aspergillosis

There are several forms of aspergillosis, including :

a. Invasive pulmonary aspergillosis

- **Description**: Serious infection that develops rapidly in immunocompromised individuals.
- **Symptoms**: Cough, chest pain, fever and breathing difficulties.

b. Allergic aspergillosis

- **Description**: allergic reaction to the presence of *Aspergillus* spores in the environment.
- **Symptoms**: Cough, shortness of breath and chronic sinusitis.

c. Aspergilloma

- **Description**: fungal mass that forms in lung cavities, often in damaged lungs.
- **Symptoms**: Cough, hemoptysis (coughing up blood) and chest pain.

3. Transmission

- **Inhalation**: Transmission is mainly by inhalation of fungal spores present in the environment, notably in soils, organic debris and decomposing materials.

- **Risk factors**: People with weakened immune systems (such as cancer patients, HIV/AIDS sufferers, or those on immunosuppressive therapy) are particularly vulnerable.

4. Diagnosis

Diagnosis of aspergillosis is based on several methods:

- **Medical imaging**: chest CT to visualize lung lesions.
- **Laboratory tests** :
  - Culture of respiratory secretions to identify *Aspergillus*.
  - Blood tests to detect specific antibodies or antigens.

5. Prevention

- **Avoiding exposure to spores**: Reduce exposure to high-risk environments, such as construction sites or areas with mold.
- **Hygiene**: Maintain good hygiene in healthcare environments to reduce the risk of infections.
- **Patient education**: Making immunocompromised patients aware of the risks of aspergillosis.

6. Treatment

- **Antifungals** :
  - **Amphotericin B**: Used to treat invasive forms of aspergillosis.
  - **Voriconazole**: Drug of choice for invasive pulmonary aspergillosis.
- **Surgery**: In some cases, surgery may be required to remove fungal masses (aspergillomas) or infected tissue.
-

7. Global Impact

- **Prevalence**: Aspergillosis is common worldwide, but particularly affects immunocompromised individuals and those with underlying lung disease.
- **Public health**: Although often treatable, invasive aspergillosis can be fatal if not diagnosed and treated promptly.

8. Conclusion

Aspergillosis is a serious fungal infection that requires special attention, especially in at-risk populations. Awareness of risk factors, good hygiene and early diagnosis are essential to prevent and treat this infection. Appropriate and prompt treatment can dramatically improve patient outcomes.

Dermatophytosis: Overview and Key Aspects

1. What is Dermatophytosis?

Dermatophytosis, commonly known as ringworm, is a skin infection caused by fungi called dermatophytes. These fungi affect the skin, hair and nails, causing a variety of skin symptoms.

2. Pathogens

The main dermatophyte genera responsible for dermatophytosis include :

- **Trichophyton**
- **Microsporum**
- **Epidermophyton**

3. Transmission

Dermatophytosis is spread mainly by :

- **Direct contact**: Contagion through contact with an infected person or animal, such as cats and dogs.
- **Contaminated objects**: Use of infected hats, towels or clothing.
- **Environment**: Exposure to contaminated surfaces, such as public showers or swimming pools.

4. Types of Dermatophytosis

Dermatophytic infections can take several forms:

a. Tinea Corporis

- **Description**: Skin infection on the body.
- **Symptoms**: Red, scaly patches with raised edges.

b. Tinea Pedis (athlete's foot)

- **Description**: Foot infection.
- **Symptoms**: Itching, redness and scaling, often between the toes.

c. Tinea Cruris (Boils)

- **Description**: groin infection.
- **Symptoms**: Itching, reddish rash and desquamation.

d. Tinea Capitis

- **Description**: Scalp infection.
- **Symptoms**: Hair loss, itching and scaly lesions.

e. Onychomycosis

- **Description**: Nail infection.
- **Symptoms**: Nail color changes, thickening and deformation.

5. Diagnosis

The diagnosis of dermatophytosis is based on several methods:

- **Clinical examination**: Assessment of symptoms and medical history.
- **Laboratory tests** :
  - **KOH**: Preparation of skin or nails with a KOH solution to examine fungal filaments.
  - **Culture**: Culture of samples to identify the fungus responsible.

6. Prevention

- **Hygiene**: Maintain good personal hygiene and keep skin dry and clean.
- **Avoid contact**: Limit contact with infected people or animals.
- **Clothing and footwear**: Use clothing and footwear made of breathable materials, and avoid sharing personal items.

7. Treatment

- **Antifungals** :
  - **Topicals**: Antifungal creams or ointments for mild infections.
  - **Oral**: Oral antifungal drugs (such as terbinafine or fluconazole) for more serious or recurrent infections.
- **Supportive care**: management of symptoms and risk factors, including humidity control.

8. Global Impact

- **Prevalence**: Dermatophytosis is widespread throughout the world, affecting millions of people, particularly in hot, humid climates.
- **Public health**: Although generally benign, it can cause discomfort and complications if left untreated.

9. Conclusion

Dermatophytosis is a common and preventable fungal infection. Awareness of risk factors, hygiene, and the importance of appropriate treatment is essential to prevent this infection. Early diagnosis and appropriate treatment can improve outcomes and reduce the spread of infection.

1.1.2.2. According to Transmission Mode

- **Zoonoses transmitted by direct contact** :
  - Transmission by contact with infected animals.
  - Examples: rabies, leptospirosis.
- **Vector-borne zoonoses** :
  - Transmission by insect vectors.
  - Examples: dengue fever, malaria, Lyme disease.
- **Foodborne zoonoses** :
  - Transmission through consumption of contaminated food.
  - Examples: salmonellosis, campylobacteriosis.
- **Environmental zoonoses** :
  - Transmission via water, soil or the environment.
  - Examples: leptospirosis, cryptosporidiosis.

1.1.2.3. According to the severity of the disease

- **Benign zoonoses** :

- Generally non-serious, often self-limiting diseases.
- Examples: certain forms of gastroenteritis.

- **Severe zoonoses** :
  - Diseases that can lead to severe complications or death.
  - Examples: rabies, viral hemorrhagic fever, tuberculosis, etc.

1.1.2.4. According to Prevalence

- **Endemic zoonoses** :
  - Consistently present in a population or region.
  - Examples: toxoplasmosis, leptospirosis in certain tropical regions.
- **Epidemic zoonoses** :
  - Sudden and rapid appearance of cases above normal levels in a population.
  - Examples: bird flu epidemics.

We need to be aware that classifying zoonoses enables us to better understand their diversity and the challenges they pose for public health. By identifying the different categories of zoonoses, researchers and health professionals can develop appropriate prevention and control strategies, helping to reduce their impact on human and animal health.

1.2. History of Zoonoses

The history of zoonoses is rich and complex, marked by significant events that have influenced public health, medicine and human-animal interactions. Key moments in the evolution of zoonoses are :

1.2.1. Antiquity and the Middle Ages

- **Antiquity**: The earliest mentions of diseases of animal origin can be found in ancient texts, such as those by Hippocrates and Galen, which refer to infections transmitted by animals. Epidemics such as the plague were often associated with rodents.
- **Middle Ages**: The Black Death (1347-1351) had a profound impact on Europe, caused by the bacterium *Yersinia pestis*, spread by fleas on rats. This event

highlighted the link between animals, vectors and the transmission of infectious diseases.

1.2.2. Renaissance and Modern

- **17th-18th centuries**: Exploration and colonization brought human populations into contact with wild animals, increasing the risk of zoonosis transmission. Epidemics of diseases such as smallpox and influenza were observed in Amerindian populations after contact with Europeans.
- **19th century**: The discovery of pathogens by scientists like Louis Pasteur was revolutionary. Pasteur developed the first vaccine against rabies, a viral zoonosis transmitted by carnivorous animals.[54]

20th century

- **Notable epidemics**: The 20th century saw the emergence of several important zoonoses, such as avian influenza (H5N1) and the Ebola virus. In 1976, the Ebola epidemic in the Democratic Republic of Congo highlighted interspecies transmission between bats and humans.
- **Advances in public health**: The development of vaccines and antibiotics has led to better control of certain zoonoses. However, globalization, urbanization and environmental change have created new opportunities for the emergence of new diseases.

21st century

- **Emergence of new zoonoses**: The COVID-19 pandemic, caused by SARS-CoV-2, illustrated the ability of zoonoses to provoke global health crises. Studies suggest that the virus probably originates from zoonotic transmission, underlining the importance of enhanced zoonosis surveillance.
- **One Health approach**: The growing recognition of the One Health approach, which links human, animal and

[54] Center for Disease Control and Prevention. (2004). The Impact of Malaria, a Leading Cause of Death Worldwide. Accessed February 27, 2006 at www.cdc.gov/malaria/ impact/index.htm

environmental health, has become essential to tackling the challenges posed by zoonoses in an interconnected world.

This history of zoonoses highlights the complex dynamics between humans, animals and environments. As we continue to face new health challenges, understanding this history is crucial to developing effective strategies for preventing and controlling zoonoses in the future. Lessons from the past can guide us in the fight against emerging and re-emerging threats to health.

1.3. Zoonosis transmission mechanisms

Zoonoses can be transmitted by a variety of mechanisms, depending on the nature of the pathogen and the interactions between humans, animals and the environment. Here are the main transmission mechanisms:

1.3.1. Direct Drive

- **Direct contact**: This involves physical contact with an infected animal or its bodily fluids (saliva, urine, excrement, blood).
  - **Examples**: Rabies is transmitted by the bite of an infected animal. Leptospirosis can be contracted through contact with the urine of infected animals.

1.3.2. Indirect transmission

- **Vectors**: Insects or other animals transmit the pathogen from one host to another. Vectors play a crucial role in the spread of many zoonoses.
  - **Examples**: Lyme disease is transmitted by ticks, while the West Nile virus is transmitted by mosquitoes.
- **Environment**: Pathogens can survive in the environment (soil, water, food) and infect humans through ingestion or contact.
  - **Examples**: Salmonellosis is often transmitted by eating contaminated food, while cryptosporidiosis can be contracted through contaminated water.

1.3.3. Food Transmission

- **Food contamination** : Foodborne zoonoses result from the ingestion of food contaminated with pathogens of animal origin.
    - **Examples**: Campylobacteriosis and salmonellosis are common in undercooked or unpasteurized meat, eggs and dairy products.

1.3.4. Animal Contact Transmission

- **Animal handling**: People working with animals (breeders, veterinarians) are often exposed to zoonoses through direct contact or medical procedures.
    - **Examples**: Brucellosis can be transmitted to farm workers when handling infected animals.

1.3.5. Airborne transmission

- **Aerosols**: Some pathogens can be transmitted by air, either by inhalation of infectious particles or by contact with contaminated surfaces.
    - **Examples**: Avian flu and bovine tuberculosis can be spread by the respiratory route.

1.3.6. Vertical transmission

- **Mother-to-child transmission**: Some zoonoses can be transmitted from mother to child during pregnancy, childbirth or breastfeeding.
    - **Examples**: Toxoplasmosis can be transmitted from mother to child, leading to serious complications.

Namely, understanding the transmission mechanisms of zoonoses is essential for developing effective prevention and control strategies. By identifying the routes by which pathogens spread, public health professionals can better target their interventions, protect human and animal populations, and reduce the risk of epidemics.

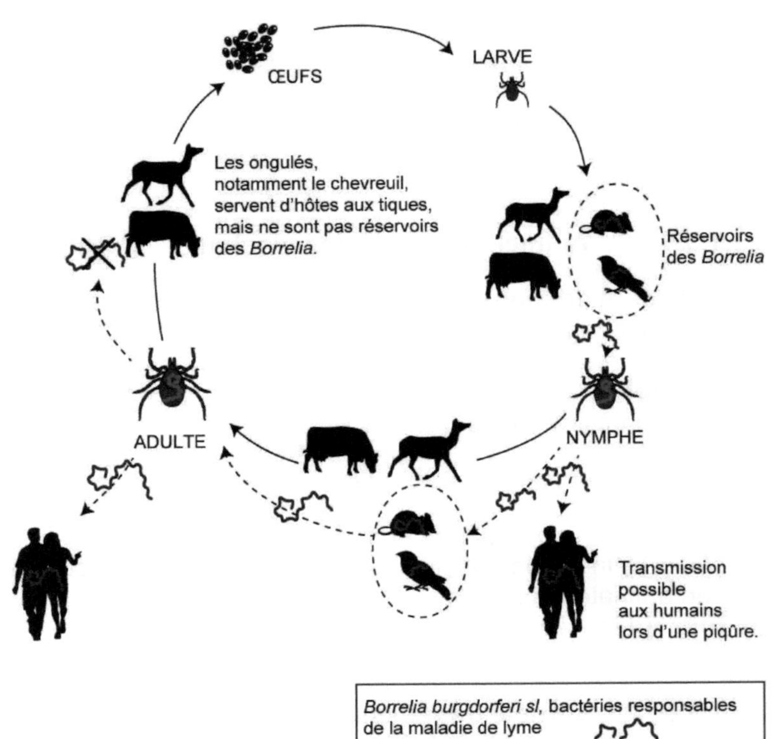
ŒUFS
LARVE
Les ongulés,
notamment le chevreuil,
servent d'hôtes aux tiques,
mais ne sont pas réservoirs
des *Borrelia*.
Réservoirs
des *Borrelia*
ADULTE
NYMPHE
Transmission
possible
aux humains
lors d'une piqûre.
Borrelia burgdorferi sl, bactéries responsables
de la maladie de lyme
Cycle de développement de la tique
Transmission des *Borrelia*

CHAPTER 2: MAIN ZOONOSES AND THEIR IMPACT

2.1 Viral zoonoses

Viral zoonoses are infections caused by viruses that can be transmitted from animals to humans. These diseases can have serious consequences for public health, and are often difficult to control due to their ability to spread rapidly. Here's an overview of two significant viral zoonoses: rabies and avian flu.

2.1.1. Rage

Pathogen

- **Virus**: Rabies virus, belonging to the Lyssavirus family.

Transmission modes

- **Transmission**: Mainly through the bite of an infected animal (often dogs). The infected animal's saliva contains the virus.

Symptoms

- **Initial phase**: fever, headache, fatigue.
- **Advanced phase**: Anxiety, confusion, hallucinations, hydrophobia, paralysis, and ultimately death if untreated.

Prevention and Control

- **Vaccination**: Vaccination of pets (especially dogs) and at-risk populations (veterinarians, travellers to high-risk areas).
- **Stray animal control**: Sterilization and vaccination programs for stray animals.

2.1.2. Avian flu

Pathogen

- **Virus**: Avian flu virus, mainly type A (H5N1, H7N9, etc.).

Transmission modes

- **Transmission**: Direct contact with infected birds (domestic or wild), their droppings or contaminated surfaces. Human-to-human transmission is rare but possible.

Symptoms

- **Human symptoms**: fever, cough, sore throat, muscle aches. In severe cases, it can lead to pneumonia and death.[55]

Prevention and Control

- **Surveillance**: Monitoring of bird populations for viral strains.
- **Poultry vaccination**: Vaccination of domestic birds in high-risk areas.
- **Education**: Raising awareness of good hygiene and biosecurity practices among at-risk populations, especially poultry farmers.

Viral zoonoses such as rabies and avian flu underline the importance of surveillance, prevention and education to protect public health. Concerted efforts are needed to control these diseases, integrating "One Health" approaches that link human, animal and environmental health. Vaccination, research and awareness-raising are key tools in the fight against these viral zoonoses.

2.2 Bacterial Zoonoses

Bacterial zoonoses are infections caused by bacteria that can be transmitted from animals to humans. These diseases can cause symptoms ranging from mild to severe, and some can lead to epidemics. Here's an overview of two

[55] Government of Quebec (2005a). An Act respecting medical laboratories, the preservation of organs, tissues, gametes and embryos and the disposal of cadavers. Accessible November 12, 2005 at www2.publicationsduquebec.gouv.qc.ca/ dynamicSearch/telecharge. php?type=2&file=/ L_0_2/L0_2.html

important bacterial zoonoses: leptospirosis and Lyme disease.[56]

2.2.1. Leptospirosis

Pathogen

- **Bacteria**: *Leptospira*, a genus of spiral-shaped bacteria.

Transmission modes

- **Transmission**: Mainly through contact with water or soil contaminated by the urine of infected animals (often rodents).
- **Routes of entry**: Bacteria enter the body through cuts, abrasions or mucous membranes.

Symptoms

- **Initial phase**: fever, headache, muscle pain, chills.
- **Advanced phase**: May develop into severe complications, including kidney, liver or lung damage (Weil syndrome).

Prevention and Control

- **Hygiene**: Avoid areas where water is contaminated, wear protective clothing.
- **Vaccination**: Vaccination of animals (especially dogs) in high-risk areas.

2.2.2. Lyme disease

Pathogen

- **Bacterium**: *Borrelia burgdorferi*, a spirochete.

Transmission modes

- **Transmission**: Mainly through the bites of infected ticks (notably the deer tick, *Ixodes scapularis*).

---

[56] Giguère, M. (2005). The health impacts of heat waves and the urban heat island effect: A review of current adaptation initiatives in Quebec. Essay submitted for Master's degree in Environment, Université de Sherbrooke, 57 pages and appendices.

- **Reservoir hosts**: Rodents and birds play a crucial role in the transmission cycle.

Symptoms

- **Initial phase**: Characteristic "target-like" rash (erythema migrans), fever, fatigue, muscle pain.
- **Advanced phase**: May lead to neurological, cardiac or joint complications if left untreated.

Prevention and Control

- **Prevention**: Use tick repellents, wear long clothing when hiking in the forest, inspect skin after outdoor activities.
- **Treatment**: Effective antibiotics, particularly doxycycline, for early infections.

Bacterial zoonoses such as leptospirosis and Lyme disease underline the importance of public health vigilance. Understanding modes of transmission, symptoms and preventive measures is essential to reduce the risk of infection and protect human and animal health.

2.3 Parasitic Zoonoses

Parasitic zoonoses are infections caused by parasites that can be transmitted from animals to humans. These diseases vary in severity and symptoms, and can be transmitted by direct contact, ingestion or vectors. Here's an overview of two important parasitic zoonoses: toxoplasmosis and echinococcosis.

1. Toxoplasmosis

Pathogen

- **Parasite**: *Toxoplasma gondii*, an intracellular protozoan.

Transmission modes

- **Transmission** :
  - Ingestion of oocysts present in the feces of infected cats.
  - Consumption of raw or undercooked meat containing cysts.

- Vertical transmission from mother to child during pregnancy.

Symptoms

- **Symptoms in adults**: Often asymptomatic, but can cause flu-like symptoms (fever, muscle aches).
- **Symptoms in the immunocompromised**: Can lead to serious complications, including brain infections.
- **Risks for the fetus**: congenital malformations and neurological problems if the mother is infected during pregnancy.[57]

Prevention and Control

- **Hygiene**: Wash hands after handling food, avoid contact with cat feces.
- **Cooking**: Cook meat properly and avoid unwashed food.

2. Echinococcosis

Pathogen

- **Parasites**: *Echinococcus granulosus* and *Echinococcus multilocularis*, cestodes (flatworms).

Transmission modes

- **Transmission** :
  - Ingestion of oocysts in water or food contaminated with dog (for *E. granulosus*) or fox (for *E. multilocularis*) feces.
  - Contact with infected animals.

Symptoms

- **Cystic echinococcosis**: formation of cysts in the liver, lungs or other organs, leading to abdominal pain, nausea and serious complications.

---

[57] Héma-Québec (2005b). Info, Newsletter for volunteers, blood donors and partners. Available February 28, 2006 at www.hema-quebec.qc.ca/media/ english/publications/ infohq_aut05eng.pdf

- **Alveolar echinococcosis**: A more aggressive, cancer-like infection that can lead to severe liver damage.[58]

Prevention and Control

- **Hygiene**: Wash hands after handling animals, avoid consuming potentially contaminated food or water.
- **Education**: Raising awareness of risks and prevention measures, particularly among dog owners.

Impact of Zoonoses on Public Health and Health Systems

Zoonoses represent a significant threat to global public health. Their impact spans several dimensions, affecting not only human health, but also healthcare systems and economies. Here is an analysis of the main impacts of zoonoses.

1. Morbidity and mortality

- **Epidemics and pandemics**: Zoonoses can lead to local epidemics or global pandemics, as demonstrated by the COVID-19 pandemic. Diseases such as rabies, avian flu and Ebola have also caused considerable loss of life.
- **Burden of disease**: Zoonoses can lead to serious illness and complications, increasing the burden on healthcare systems. This applies not only to acute cases, but also to chronic complications associated with certain infections.

2. Economic costs

- **Healthcare costs**: Medical care to treat zoonotic infections increases healthcare expenditure. Hospitalization, treatment and long-term care for complications can weigh heavily on public health budgets.
- **Impact on agriculture**: Zoonoses affect animal productivity, leading to economic losses in the agricultural sector. Epidemics can lead to quarantines, destruction of

[58] Haines A., McMichael, A.J. & Epstein, P.R. (2000). Environment and health: 2. Global climate change and health. JAMC;163(6):729-34.

infected animals and restrictions on trade in animal products.[59]

3. Pressure on healthcare systems

- **Surveillance and Response**: Zoonoses require robust health systems to monitor, detect and respond rapidly to outbreaks. This requires significant human and financial resources, which are often limited in low- and middle-income countries.
- **Interdisciplinary coordination**: Managing zoonoses requires collaboration between various sectors (public health, veterinary medicine, environment). The absence of such cooperation can lead to ineffective responses and delays in the management of health crises.

4. Education and awareness

- **Public awareness**: Zoonoses underline the importance of education and community awareness. Informing the public about modes of transmission and prevention measures is crucial to limiting the spread of disease.
- **Training health professionals**: Health and animal health professionals need to be trained to identify and treat zoonoses, which requires ongoing training programs.

5. Behavioral changes

- **Health practices**: Zoonosis epidemics can lead to changes in health-related behaviors, whether in farming, food or hygiene practices. These changes can have lasting effects on public health.

The impact of zoonoses on public health and healthcare systems is vast and interconnected. To mitigate these impacts, it is essential to adopt integrated approaches, such as the One Health model, which recognizes the interdependence between human, animal

---

[59] MacLean, J.D., Demers, A.-M., Ndao, M., Kokoskin, E., Ward, B.J. & Gyorkos, T.W. (2004). Malaria epidemics and surveillance systems in Canada. Emerg Infect Dis;10 (7) : 1195- 1201.

and environmental health. By strengthening surveillance, improving communication and investing in resilient health systems, we can better prepare our societies to face the challenges posed by zoonoses.

CHAPTER 3: RISK FACTORS AND VULNERABILITY

3.1 Human-Animal Interactions

Interactions between humans and animals are complex and varied, playing a crucial role in the transmission of zoonoses. These interactions can be influenced by cultural, environmental, economic and behavioral factors. Here's an overview of the main dimensions of these interactions and their impact on public health.

1.types of interaction

a. Pets

- **Livestock**: Livestock (cattle, pigs, poultry) are often in close contact with humans. Farming practices can encourage the transmission of zoonoses such as salmonellosis and brucellosis.
- **Pets**: Dogs, cats and other pets can transmit zoonoses such as toxoplasmosis or rabies through direct or indirect contact.

b. Wild animals

- **Contact with wildlife**: Human activities such as hunting, fishing and tourism increase interactions with wild animals, which can lead to zoonotic transmissions (e.g. Ebola virus).
- **Shared habitat**: The destruction of natural habitats by urbanization or agriculture is leading to increased proximity between humans and wildlife, increasing the risk of disease transmission.

3.2 Factors Contributing to Interactions

a. Environmental changes

- **Urbanization**: the growth of cities and the expansion of urban areas are leading to a reduction in natural spaces, forcing wild animals to adapt and cohabit with humans.

- **Climate change**: Climate change can influence animal migrations and the distribution of zoonoses, modifying interactions between species.

b. Cultural and economic practices

- **Eating habits**: Some cultures consume wild animals or practice specific animal husbandry practices, increasing the risk of zoonoses (e.g. bushmeat consumption).
- **Intensive rearing**: Industrial rearing methods can create conditions conducive to the emergence of zoonoses, favoring the rapid spread of pathogens.[60]

3.3 Public health implications

a. ***Disease surveillance***

- **Importance of Surveillance**: Close monitoring of human-animal interactions is essential to detect and control zoonoses. This includes monitoring animal populations and human outbreaks.
- **Interdisciplinary collaboration**: Human and animal health professionals need to work together to share information and coordinate surveillance efforts.

b. Education and awareness

- **Informativeness**: Raising public awareness of the risks associated with interactions with animals, particularly in rural or at-risk areas, is crucial to preventing the transmission of zoonoses.
- **Training professionals**: Veterinarians, farmers and others need to be trained to recognize the signs of zoonoses and implement effective prevention practices.

Human-animal interactions are an essential facet of public health, particularly when it comes to zoonoses. Understanding these interactions and the factors that influence them is crucial to developing effective prevention and control strategies. By adopting an integrated approach,

---

[60] Ministère de l'Agriculture, des Pêcheries et de l'Alimentation du Québec (2006a). Surveillance de la santé animale. Available online June 28, 2006 at www.mapaq.gouv.qc.ca/ Fr/Productions/ santeanimale/surveillance/

taking into account human, animal and environmental dimensions, we can better protect the health of populations and reduce the risk of zoonotic disease transmission.

3.4. Environmental and climatic factors affecting zoonoses

Environmental and climatic factors play a crucial role in the emergence and spread of zoonoses. These factors influence pathogen distribution, animal population dynamics, and human-animal interactions. Here's an overview of the main factors contributing to this problem.

1. Climate change

a. Temperature

- **Influence on vectors**: Temperature variations can affect the reproduction and survival of vectors such as mosquitoes and ticks, increasing the risk of transmission of diseases such as malaria and Lyme disease.
- **Disease distribution**: Global warming can enable certain zoonoses to spread to new regions, where environmental conditions become favorable.

b. Precipitation

- **Flooding and Risk of Transmission**: Extreme weather events, such as floods, can contaminate drinking water sources with pathogens, increasing the risk of waterborne diseases such as leptospirosis.
- **Vector habitats**: Changes in precipitation patterns can alter vector habitats, favoring the transmission of zoonoses.

3.5. Habitat and ecosystems

a. Deforestation

- **Ecosystem disruption**: The destruction of natural habitats through deforestation increases interactions between wild animals and humans, facilitating the transmission of zoonoses such as the Ebola virus.

- **Biodiversity loss**: Reduced biodiversity can affect ecosystems and increase the resilience of pathogens, making epidemics more likely.

b. Urbanization

- **Proximity to wildlife**: Urbanization is leading to increased proximity between human populations and wild animals, creating opportunities for the transmission of zoonotic diseases.
- **Poor waste management**: inadequate waste management can attract rodents and other animals carrying zoonoses, increasing the risk of infection.

3.6. Farming practices

a. Intensive breeding

- **Conditions conducive to transmission**: Intensive livestock farming practices favor the rapid spread of pathogens due to high animal density and often unsanitary living conditions.
- **Antibiotic resistance**: Excessive use of antibiotics in livestock farming can contribute to the development of resistant strains, making it more difficult to treat zoonotic infections.

b. Agriculture and the food system

- **Food contamination**: Unsustainable agricultural practices can lead to food contamination by pathogens, increasing the risk of foodborne zoonoses such as salmonellosis.

3.7. Monitoring and preparation

a. Importance of Environmental Monitoring

- **Ecosystem monitoring**: Monitoring ecosystems and animal populations can help identify emerging zoonotic risks.
- **Risk modeling**: Using climate and epidemiological models to predict changes in the distribution of zoonoses can help anticipate and prepare appropriate responses.

Environmental and climatic factors are interdependent and play a significant role in the dynamics of zoonoses. Understanding these interactions is essential for developing effective prevention and control strategies. An integrated approach that takes into account environmental, climatic and human health aspects is essential to reduce the risk of zoonosis transmission and protect public health.

3.8. The role of farming and livestock practices in zoonoses

Agricultural and animal husbandry practices play a crucial role in the emergence, transmission and spread of zoonoses. These activities influence not only animal and human health, but also the environment. Here's an overview of the different aspects of this role.

1. Livestock intensification

a. Animal living conditions

- **High density**: Intensive livestock production systems, characterized by high animal density, favor the rapid spread of pathogens. Infections can spread rapidly through herds, increasing the risk of transmission to humans.
- **Stress and disease**: Animals raised under stressful conditions are more likely to develop diseases, which can increase the virulence of pathogens.

b. Use of antibiotics

- **Antibiotic resistance**: Excessive use of antibiotics to prevent disease or promote growth can lead to the development of resistant bacterial strains, making the treatment of zoonotic infections more difficult.

3.9. Farming practices

a. Food contamination

- **Handling and processing**: Food handling and processing practices can introduce pathogens into the food chain. For example, contact between contaminated animal products and plant foods can lead to foodborne zoonoses.

- **Irrigation and water**: Inadequate management of water resources for irrigation can contaminate crops with pathogens, increasing the risk of food-borne diseases.

b. Waste management

- **Animal waste**: The accumulation of animal waste on farms can encourage the proliferation of pathogens and attract vectors such as rodents and insects, increasing the risk of transmission.

3.10. Interaction with wildlife

a. Contact with wild animals

- **Inter-species transmission**: Farming practices that encourage contact between domestic animals and wildlife can facilitate the transmission of zoonoses. For example, rodents can transmit leptospirosis to farm animals and, by extension, to humans.
- **Habitat Modified**: The expansion of farmland is altering natural habitats, increasing interactions between humans, domestic animals and wildlife.

3.11. Awareness-raising and education

a. Prevention practices

- **Farmer training**: Training in best animal health and food safety practices is essential to reduce the risk of zoonoses. This includes waste management, hygiene and disease surveillance.
- **Raising public awareness**: Informing consumers about the risks associated with animal products and farming practices can help reduce the transmission of zoonoses.

3.12. Sustainable approaches

a. Ecological agriculture

- **Sustainable practices**: Adopting sustainable agricultural practices, such as organic farming and crop rotation, can reduce the risk of zoonoses by promoting biodiversity and limiting the use of antibiotics.

- **Integrated management**: An integrated approach combining animal health, human health and environmental protection (One Health model) is essential to prevent zoonoses.

Farming and breeding practices have a significant impact on the dynamics of zoonoses. By adopting sustainable practices, raising farmers' awareness and improving resource management, it is possible to reduce the risk of zoonosis transmission and protect public health. An integrated approach is crucial to tackling this complex and interconnected issue.

CHAPTER 4: ZOONOSIS MONITORING AND DETECTION

4.1. Existing surveillance systems for zoonoses

Zoonosis surveillance is essential to detect, control and prevent the emergence of infectious diseases of animal origin. Several monitoring systems have been set up at different levels, ranging from local initiatives to international programs. Here's an overview of the main existing surveillance systems.

1. National surveillance

a. Health surveillance systems

- **Public health systems**: Many countries have surveillance systems for communicable diseases that include zoonoses. These systems collect and analyze data on human and animal cases, facilitating early detection of epidemics.
- **Epidemiological vigilance**: Public health agencies monitor zoonosis trends and alert health authorities to any increase in cases.

b. Veterinary surveillance

- **Animal surveillance programs**: Ministries of Agriculture or Animal Health set up surveillance programs to detect animal diseases such as brucellosis, bovine tuberculosis and avian influenza.
- **Disease reporting**: Veterinarians are often required to report cases of zoonotic diseases, enabling a rapid response to epidemics.

4.2. International monitoring

a. World Health Organization (WHO)

- **Alert and Response System**: WHO monitors zoonotic disease outbreaks worldwide and works with countries to share information and implement coordinated responses.

b. World Organization for Animal Health (OIE)

- **Notification system**: The OIE has established an animal disease notification framework, where countries report outbreaks of zoonoses and other animal diseases. This makes it possible to monitor the distribution and impact of diseases worldwide.

c. Food and Agriculture Organization (FAO)

- **Food Surveillance Programs**: FAO works on programs to monitor food-borne zoonoses and promote food safety practices.

4.3. Integrated Monitoring Systems

a. One Health approach

- **Interdisciplinary collaboration**: Increasingly, surveillance systems are adopting a One Health approach, integrating data on human, animal and environmental health. This enables a better understanding of the interactions between these fields, and facilitates a more effective response to zoonoses.

b. Monitoring networks

- **Regional networks**: Networks such as the European Network for Disease Surveillance (ECDC) and the Global Network for Disease Surveillance (GMOS) facilitate information sharing and collaboration between countries to monitor and respond to zoonoses.

4.4. Monitoring through Technology

a. Big Data and Artificial Intelligence

- **Data analysis**: The use of artificial intelligence and big data analytics makes it possible to process large quantities of information to detect epidemic trends and predict the risk of zoonoses.
- **Mobile applications**: Applications and online platforms enable rapid reporting of disease cases, facilitating real-time data collection.

b. Genomic surveillance

- **Genome sequencing**: Sequencing viral and bacterial genomes helps track the evolution of pathogens and identify the strains responsible for epidemics.

Zoonosis monitoring systems are essential for protecting public health and controlling epidemics. The integration of human, animal and environmental surveillance efforts, and the adoption of new technologies, enhance the ability to detect, prevent and control zoonoses effectively. International and interdisciplinary collaboration is essential to meet this complex and dynamic challenge.

4.5. Emerging technologies for detecting zoonoses

The emergence of new technologies has considerably improved the ability to detect zoonoses quickly and efficiently. These innovations enable more accurate surveillance, rapid response to epidemics and a better understanding of disease dynamics. Here's an overview of emerging technologies in this field.[61]

1. Genomic sequencing

- **New Generation Sequencing (NGS)**: This technique enables the rapid sequencing of pathogen genomes, facilitating strain identification, mutation tracking and disease transmission analysis.
- **Epidemiological surveillance**: Genomic sequencing helps track epidemics by providing information on the origin and spread of pathogens.

2. Rapid diagnostic tests

- **Early Detection Tests**: PCR (polymerase chain reaction)-based tests enable rapid, accurate detection of pathogens in clinical or environmental samples.

[61] Ministère de l'Agriculture, des Pêcheries et de l'Alimentation du Québec (2006b). Avian influenza. Accessible online June 28, 2006 at www.mapaq.gouv.qc.ca/Fr/Productions/ santeanimale/surveillance/maladies animales/grippeaviaire

- **Antigenic tests**: These tests are designed to detect specific proteins in pathogens and can provide results within minutes, which is crucial during epidemics.

4.6. Environmental Monitoring Technologies

- **IoT sensors and devices**: Environmental sensors, integrated into IoT (Internet of Things) networks, monitor environmental conditions conducive to the transmission of zoonoses (e.g. temperature, humidity).
- **Drones and remote sensing**: Drones can be used to monitor wildlife habitats, enabling wildlife data to be collected and zoonosis risks to be identified.

4.7. Modeling and Big Data

- **Big Data analysis**: Using large quantities of data from a variety of sources (clinical, environmental, demographic), we can identify trends and risks of zoonoses.
- **Predictive modeling**: Mathematical and statistical models help predict the emergence of zoonoses by analyzing interactions between environmental factors and animal and human populations.

4.8. Mobile Applications and Digital Platforms

- **Real-time reporting**: Mobile applications enable healthcare professionals and the public to quickly report suspected cases of zoonoses, facilitating a rapid response.
- **Collaborative databases**: online platforms centralize data on zoonoses, enabling information to be shared between researchers, health professionals and health authorities.

4.9. High-definition sequencing technologies

- **Metagenomic sequencing**: This technique makes it possible to analyze complex samples (such as environmental samples) to identify several pathogens simultaneously.
- **Real-time sequencing**: This method enables sequencing to be carried out in the field, providing almost instantaneous results for rapid intervention.

Emerging technologies in zoonosis detection offer powerful tools for improving the surveillance, prevention and control of infectious diseases of animal origin. By integrating these technologies into public health and veterinary systems, it is possible to strengthen resilience to zoonotic threats and protect human and animal health. Interdisciplinary and international collaboration will be essential to maximize the impact of these innovations.

410 The Importance of Interdisciplinary Collaboration in Zoonosis Control

The fight against zoonoses requires an integrated approach that combines the expertise of several disciplines. Interdisciplinary collaboration is crucial to improving epidemic prevention, detection and response. Here are the main reasons why collaboration is so important.[62]

1. One Health approach

- **One Health concept**: This concept recognizes that human, animal and environmental health are interconnected. A One Health approach makes it possible to understand the complex interactions between these fields and to develop effective public health strategies.
- **Coordination of Efforts**: By bringing together human, veterinary and environmental health professionals, we can better manage zoonoses that emerge from wildlife, domestic animals and the environment.

2. Improved monitoring and detection

- **Information sharing** : Collaboration between the public health, animal health and ecology sectors enables information sharing that is crucial to zoonosis surveillance.

---

[62] Ogden, N.H., Maarouf, A., Barker, I.K., Bigras-Poulin, M., Lindsay, L.R., Morshed, M.G.,
O'Callaghan, C.J., Ramay, F., Waltner-Toews, D., Charron, D.F. Climate change and the
potential for range expansion of the Lyme disease vector Ixodes scapularis in Canada.
Int J Parasitol. 2006 Jan;36(1):63–70.

- **Integrated Surveillance Systems**: Surveillance systems that integrate data from a variety of disciplines enable earlier detection of disease outbreaks and proactive response.

3. Research & Development

- **Joint Innovation**: Interdisciplinary teams can conduct more comprehensive and innovative research, combining expertise in medicine, biology, ecology and the social sciences.
- **Developing Solutions**: Collaboration between researchers, practitioners and decision-makers helps develop practical solutions tailored to local needs.

4. Rapid Response to Epidemics

- **Crisis coordination**: In the event of an epidemic, rapid response requires coordination between different players, including health agencies, non-governmental organizations and local communities.
- **Resource mobilization**: Collaboration enables resources to be better mobilized and ensures an effective response, minimizing the impact of zoonoses on public health.

5. Awareness and education

- **Interdisciplinary training**: Joint training of human and animal health professionals facilitates understanding of zoonoses and best prevention practices.
- **Community awareness**: Awareness campaigns that integrate human, animal and environmental health perspectives are more effective in informing the public about risks and prevention measures.

6. Sustainable Policies and Practices

- **Policy-making**: Decision-makers who work with experts from different disciplines can develop more effective and sustainable policies for public health and natural resource management.[63]

---

[63] Health Canada (2005). Your Health and a Changing Climate: Newsletter.

- **Ecological approaches**: Interdisciplinary collaboration promotes the adoption of sustainable agricultural and environmental practices, thereby reducing the risk of zoonoses.

Interdisciplinary collaboration is essential to meet the complex challenges posed by zoonoses. By integrating the perspectives and expertise of various fields, it is possible to develop holistic and effective approaches to the prevention, detection and response to infectious diseases of animal origin.[64] This contributes not only to protecting human and animal health, but also to preserving the environment, thus ensuring a healthier and more sustainable future.

4.11. Concrete examples of successful interdisciplinary collaboration in the fight against zoonoses

Interdisciplinary collaboration has led to notable successes in the prevention and management of zoonoses. Here are a few concrete examples:

1. World Health Organization (WHO) One Health Initiative

- **Background**: WHO, in collaboration with the World Organization for Animal Health (OIE) and FAO, has launched the One Health initiative to strengthen surveillance and response to zoonoses.
- **Results**: This initiative has coordinated efforts between the human, animal and environmental health sectors, facilitating early detection of diseases such as avian flu and Ebola. Participating countries have developed integrated action plans to improve resilience in the face of epidemics.

2. Response to the Ebola Epidemic in West Africa (2014-2016)

Accessible August 25, 2005 at www.c-ciarn.ca/health/app/filerepository/ 348DC2838BCB 498DB86828FA12122713.pdf

[64] Pollution probe (2004). Primer on climate change and human health.

Accessible August 25, 2005 at www.pollution probe.org/Reports/climatechange primer(en).pdf

- **Background**: The Ebola epidemic required a rapid response from a variety of disciplines, including public health, veterinary medicine, ecology and logistics.
- **Collaboration**: Interdisciplinary teams were formed, combining doctors, veterinarians, epidemiologists and humanitarian workers. This approach made it possible to identify animal reservoirs of the virus and implement effective control strategies.
- **Results**: The collaboration led to a significant reduction in virus transmission and helped to better prepare healthcare systems for future epidemics.

3. Lyme disease surveillance

- **Background**: Lyme disease is transmitted by ticks and has become a major public health concern in certain regions.
- **Collaboration**: Researchers in public health, biology, ecology and climatology worked together to understand the environmental and climatic factors influencing the spread of the disease.
- **Results**: This collaboration has made it possible to develop predictive models for the distribution of ticks and cases of Lyme disease, thus contributing to targeted prevention strategies.

4. Avian Influenza Surveillance Program in Asia

- **Background**: Asia has been the focus of several avian influenza epidemics, necessitating enhanced surveillance.
- **Collaboration**: Scientists, veterinarians, agronomists and public health officials worked together to monitor poultry populations and humans at risk.
- **Results**: This program enabled the rapid detection of avian flu outbreaks and effective intervention, thus reducing the risk of transmission to humans and the spread of the disease.

5. Animal and Public Health Initiatives in Latin America

- **Context**: Several Latin American countries have set up integrated health programs to combat zoonoses such as leptospirosis and brucellosis.
- **Collaboration**: Ministries of public health, agriculture and the environment work together to monitor cases, educate communities and implement interventions.
- **Results**: These efforts have reduced the incidence of these diseases and improved the health of rural communities, by integrating sustainable health practices.

These examples illustrate how interdisciplinary collaboration can improve the detection, prevention and management of zoonoses. By pooling skills and expertise from different fields, it is possible to create more effective solutions to the complex challenges posed by infectious diseases of animal origin. These successes underline the importance of an integrated approach to protecting human, animal and environmental health.

CHAPTER 5: PREVENTION APPROACH

5.1. Animal and Human Vaccination in Zoonosis Control

Vaccination is one of the most effective tools for preventing zoonoses in both animals and humans. It plays a crucial role in reducing disease transmission, protecting vulnerable populations and safeguarding public health. Here's an analysis of the importance of vaccination in this context.

1. Animal Vaccination

a. Importance

- **Disease prevention**: Vaccinating pets (such as dogs and cats) is essential to prevent zoonoses such as rabies, leptospirosis and Lyme disease.
- **Epidemic control**: Vaccination programs for farm animals (such as cattle and poultry) help control zoonotic diseases like brucellosis and avian influenza, reducing the risk of transmission to humans.

b. Vaccination programs

- **Rabies vaccination**: Many countries have introduced rabies vaccination programs for dogs, reducing the risk of rabies transmission to humans.
- **Livestock vaccines**: Vaccines are available for diseases such as brucellosis and bovine tuberculosis, helping to protect animal and human health.[65]

2. Vaccination of Human Populations

a. Importance

- **Protecting public health**: Vaccinating human populations is crucial to preventing zoonoses such as rabies, avian flu and yellow fever, especially in high-risk areas.

---

[65] Badin de Montjoye Th., Thorel M.F. and Garin- Bastuji B. - Trends in bovine tuberculosis in France: 2002 review and outlook. *Bull. GTV*, 2004, **23**, 311- 314.

- **Herd immunity**: Vaccinating at-risk groups (such as farm workers or veterinarians) helps establish herd immunity, limiting the spread of disease.[66]

b. Vaccination campaigns

- **Rabies vaccination**: Targeted vaccination campaigns are carried out in regions where rabies is endemic, to protect human populations and control the disease.
- **Vaccines against zoonotic diseases**: Vaccines against zoonoses such as avian flu and dengue fever are being developed and distributed, strengthening the public health response.

3. Synergy between Animal and Human Vaccination

- **Integrated approach**: A coordinated approach combining animal and human vaccination is essential to control zoonoses. For example, vaccinating dogs against rabies reduces the risk to humans, creating a beneficial synergy.
- **Education and awareness**: Raising public awareness of the importance of vaccinating animals and humans is crucial to encourage participation in vaccination programs.

4. Challenges and prospects

a. Challenges

- **Access to vaccines**: In many parts of the world, access to vaccines remains a challenge for both animals and humans.
- **Education and acceptance**: Mistrust of vaccines can undermine immunization programs, requiring awareness-raising efforts to educate the public about their benefits.

b. Outlook

- **Vaccine innovations**: The development of new vaccines, including RNA-based and multivalent vaccines, could improve the effectiveness of vaccination against zoonoses.

---

[66] Acha P.N. and Szyfres B. - Zoonoses and communicable diseases common to man and animals (Second edition). Office International des Epizooties, 1989, 1063p.

- **Strengthening health systems**: Investing in health infrastructure and integrated vaccination programs can boost resilience to zoonoses in the long term.

Vaccination of animals and human populations is a key element in the fight against zoonoses. By combining targeted vaccination efforts with educational and awareness-raising strategies, it is possible to significantly reduce the risk of transmission of infectious diseases of animal origin. An integrated and collaborative approach is essential to protect public health and improve global health security.

Community Education and Awareness in Zoonosis Control

Community education and awareness-raising are crucial elements in the prevention and control of zoonoses. By informing people about the risks, modes of transmission and preventive measures, we can significantly reduce the incidence of these diseases. Here's how these efforts can be effectively implemented.

1. The importance of education

a. Understanding Zoonoses

- **Risk awareness**: Educating communities about what zoonoses are, how they spread and their consequences for human and animal health.
- **Modes of transmission**: Provide information on modes of transmission, including contact with infected animals, consumption of contaminated food and the bite of vectors such as mosquitoes and ticks.

b. Prevention practices

- **Hygiene and Safety**: Promote personal and food hygiene practices, such as hand washing, proper cooking and animal waste management.
- **Vaccination**: Raising awareness of the importance of vaccinating pets and livestock to reduce the risk of transmission.

2. Awareness strategies

a. Awareness campaigns

- **Workshops and Seminars**: Organize workshops in schools, community centers and farms to discuss zoonoses and prevention practices.
- **Educational Material**: Distribute brochures, posters and educational videos that explain zoonoses and preventive measures in an accessible way.[67]

b. Media use

- **Social networks and local media**: Use social networks, radio and television to spread awareness of zoonoses, especially in high-risk regions.
- **Testimonials and Stories**: Share testimonials from people affected by zoonoses to humanize the message and raise awareness.[68]

3. Working with local stakeholders

a. Partnerships with health authorities

- **Involvement of local authorities**: Collaborate with local health authorities to ensure that awareness-raising messages are consistent and adapted to community needs.
- **Training Programs for Professionals**: Train community health workers, veterinarians and teachers to become ambassadors for public health.

*b. **Community involvement***

- **Discussion groups**: Create discussion groups within communities to exchange ideas and concerns about zoonoses.

---

[67] Chomel B. - Emerging bacterial zoonoses. *Point Vét*, 2000, **31**, 195- 202.
[68] Bénet J.J. and Haddad N. - Dangers, risks and prevention of zoonoses transmitted to humans by dog and cat bites. *Le Nouveau Praticien Vétérinaire*, 2004, **18**, 21-25.

- **Community initiatives**: Encourage local initiatives, such as clean-up days or animal vaccination campaigns, to strengthen community involvement.

4. Monitoring and evaluation

a. Program evaluation

- **Community feedback**: Gather feedback from participants on the effectiveness of awareness programs to adjust strategies.
- **Impact measurement**: Evaluate the impact of awareness-raising initiatives on zoonoses knowledge and preventive behaviors within communities.

Community education and awareness-raising are essential to prevent and control zoonoses. By adopting targeted, collaborative strategies, it is possible to strengthen community resilience in the face of health risks. Community involvement and collaboration with local stakeholders are key to the success of these initiatives. A well-informed community is better equipped to protect its health and that of its animals, thus contributing to overall health security.

Hygiene and Pest Control in Zoonosis Control

Hygiene and pest control are fundamental elements in the prevention of zoonoses. By maintaining clean environments and effectively managing pest populations, we can reduce the risk of transmission of infectious diseases of animal origin. Here's an overview of best practices and strategies.

1. The importance of hygiene

a. Personal hygiene

- **Hand Washing**: Frequent hand washing, especially after handling animals or animal products, is essential to prevent the transmission of zoonoses.
- **Protective equipment**: Use gloves, masks and other protective equipment when handling sick animals or animal waste.

b. Food hygiene

- **Food handling**: Ensure that foods of animal origin are properly cooked and handled under sanitary conditions. Avoid cross-contamination between raw and cooked foods.
- **Storage and preservation**: Store food at appropriate temperatures to prevent the proliferation of pathogens.

2. Pest control

a. Pest identification

- **Species Monitoring**: Identify rodents, insects and other pests that may carry zoonoses. Knowing which species are present helps to better target control efforts.
- **Risk Assessment**: Evaluate the risks associated with pests in urban, agricultural and domestic environments.

b. Control strategies

- **Preventive methods** :
  - **Exclusion**: Seal openings in buildings to prevent pests from entering.
  - **Regular cleaning**: Maintain rigorous cleaning practices to eliminate sources of food and shelter.
- **Management methods** :
  - **Biological control**: Use natural predators or specific pathogens to control pest populations.
  - **Pesticides and Rodenticides**: Use chemicals responsibly and in accordance with guidelines to avoid negative impacts on the environment.

3. Education and awareness

a. Risk awareness

- **Pest information**: Educate communities about zoonoses associated with pests, such as leptospirosis (transmitted by rodents) and Lyme disease (transmitted by ticks).
- **Preventive practices**: educate people about best practices in hygiene and pest control.

b. Community programs

- **Clean-up initiatives**: Organize community clean-up days to eliminate waste and reduce pest harborage.
- **Training workshops**: Offer workshops on pest control and hygiene for farmers and pet owners.

4. Monitoring and assessment

a. Pest control

- **Monitoring systems**: Set up monitoring systems to track pest populations and detect disease outbreaks early.
- **Community reporting**: Encourage community members to report pest infestations and problems.

b. Effort evaluation

- **Measuring Impact**: Evaluate the effectiveness of hygiene and pest control programs by monitoring the incidence of zoonoses in the community.
- **Adjusting strategies**: Use the data collected to adjust and improve control strategies.

Hygiene and pest control are essential to prevent zoonoses and protect public health. By adopting rigorous hygiene practices and effectively managing pest populations, communities can significantly reduce the risk of transmission of infectious diseases of animal origin. A collaborative approach, combining education, awareness-raising and community involvement, is key to ensuring the success of these initiatives.

CHAPTER 6: CONTROL STRATEGIES

Response to Zoonotic Outbreaks

Responding quickly and effectively to zoonotic disease outbreaks is essential to protect public, animal and environmental health. Here's an overview of the key steps and strategies involved in managing zoonotic disease outbreaks.

1. Early detection

a. Monitoring and warning system

- **Epidemiological surveillance**: Set up robust surveillance systems to rapidly detect cases of zoonoses in animals and humans.
- **Alert systems**: Use early warning systems to signal disease outbreaks and trigger a rapid response.

b. Case reporting

- **Training health professionals**: Train doctors, veterinarians and community health workers to recognize the signs of zoonoses and report suspected cases.
- **Community involvement**: Encourage the population to report cases of suspected infections.

2. Epidemiological investigation

a. Source search

- **Case analysis**: Identify potential sources of the epidemic (animals, environment, supply chains).
- **Contact study** : Track contacts of confirmed cases to limit spread.

b. Risk assessment

- **Epidemiological Modeling**: Using models to assess epidemic propagation dynamics and predict impacts.

- **Case Mapping**: Create epidemiological maps to visualize spread and target interventions.[69]

3. Intervention and Control

a. Animal control measures

- **Quarantine and isolation**: Quarantine infected animals and isolate suspected cases to prevent transmission.
- **Vaccination**: Deploy targeted vaccination campaigns to protect animals at risk and reduce transmission to humans.

b. Public health measures

- **Public awareness**: Informing communities about the risks and measures to take to protect themselves.
- **Pest control**: Implement pest control programs to reduce transmission vectors.[70]

4. Treatment and care

a. Access to healthcare

- **Case management**: Ensure rapid access to care for infected people, including specific treatment for certain zoonoses.
- **Case follow-up**: Set up a follow-up system to monitor the progress of cases and the effects of treatments.

b. Animal care

- **Veterinary Care**: Providing veterinary care for sick animals and reducing animal suffering.

5. Coordination and collaboration

[69] Hantz S. and Darde M.L. - How to prevent the risks of zoonosis for the immunocompromised subject. *Le nouveau praticien vétérinaire*, 2004, **18**, 41-43.

[70] Hahn B.H., Shaw G.M., De Cock K.M. and Sharp P.M. - AIDS as a zoonosis: scientific and public health implications. *Science*, 2000, **287**(5453), 607-614.

a. Multi-sector partnerships

- **One Health Collaboration**: Involving the human, animal and environmental health sectors for an integrated response.
- **Stakeholder engagement**: Work with NGOs, local governments and international organizations to coordinate efforts.

b. Crisis management

- **Epidemic Response Plans**: Develop and implement emergency plans to respond effectively to epidemics.
- **Crisis Communication**: Ensure clear and transparent communication with the public and the media to avoid misinformation.

6. Assessment and learning

a. Post-epidemic analysis

- **Evaluation of Responses**: Assess the effectiveness of the measures put in place and identify lessons to be learned.
- **Reports and recommendations**: Produce reports detailing responses to epidemics and make recommendations to improve future interventions.

b. Capacity building

- **Training and awareness**: Organize training courses for health professionals and communities on zoonosis management.
- **Improving infrastructure**: investing in public and veterinary health infrastructure to strengthen resilience against future epidemics.

Conclusion

Responding to zoonotic disease outbreaks requires a coordinated, integrated approach involving early detection, investigation, intervention, coordination and evaluation. By strengthening collaboration between the human, animal and environmental health sectors, it is possible to minimize the impact of zoonoses on public health and better prepare communities to cope with future epidemics.

Regulations and Public Health Policies in the Fight against Zoonoses

Public health regulations and policies play a crucial role in the prevention and control of zoonoses. They establish standards and protocols to protect human, animal and environmental health. Here's an overview of the main components and their importance.[71]

1. Regulatory framework

a. National legislation

- **Public health laws**: Many countries have specific laws governing the surveillance, prevention and control of zoonoses. These laws may include case notification requirements, mandatory vaccinations and intervention protocols.
- **Veterinary regulations**: Animal health laws set standards for the vaccination, treatment and welfare of animals, helping to reduce the risk of zoonoses.

b. International standards

- **World Health Organization (WHO)**: WHO provides recommendations and protocols for the management of zoonoses worldwide.
- **World Organization for Animal Health (OIE)**: The OIE develops international animal health standards, including guidelines for the prevention of zoonoses.

2. Public health policy

a. Prevention strategies

- **Vaccination programs**: Public health policies include vaccination programs for domestic and farm animals, aimed at reducing the transmission of zoonotic diseases.

[71] Hubalek Z. - Emerging human infectious diseases: anthroponoses, zoonoses, and sapronoses. *Emerg. Infect. Dis.* 2003; **9**(3); 403-404.

- **Monitoring and Control**: Establish monitoring systems to detect zoonoses early and implement appropriate control measures.[72]

b. Awareness-raising and education

- **Awareness campaigns**: Public policies must include education campaigns on zoonosis risks and prevention practices, targeting both rural and urban communities.
- **Training professionals**: Training programs for health professionals, veterinarians and community workers are essential to strengthen response capacity.

3. Intersectoral coordination

a. One Health approach

- **Cross-sector collaboration**: Policies must promote a One Health approach, integrating the human, animal and environmental health sectors for effective zoonosis management.
- **Public-Private Partnerships**: Establish partnerships with NGOs, universities and private companies to strengthen the response to zoonoses.

b. Epidemic Response Plans

- **Contingency plans**: Develop contingency plans to respond rapidly to zoonotic disease outbreaks, including clear protocols for detection, isolation and treatment.
- **Simulations and exercises**: Organize simulation exercises to test preparedness and coordination between the various players involved in zoonosis management.

4. Monitoring and assessment

---

[72] Haydon D.T., Cleaveland S., Taylor L.H. and Laurenson - Identifying reservoirs of infection: a conceptual and practical challenge. *Emerg. Infect. Dis.* 2002, **8**(12), 1468-1473.

a. Policy monitoring

- **Program evaluation**: Set up evaluation mechanisms to measure the effectiveness of public health policies and zoonosis prevention programs.
- **Reports and Recommendations**: Produce regular reports on the status of zoonoses, the responses implemented and recommendations for improving policies.

b. Research and Innovation

- **Support for research**: Policies should encourage research into zoonoses, including the development of new vaccines and treatments.
- **Data Sharing**: Facilitate data sharing between researchers, health agencies and policy-makers for informed decision-making.

5. Challenges and prospects

a. Challenges

- **Lack of resources**: Many countries, particularly in low-income regions, lack the resources to implement effective public health policies.
- **Public acceptance**: mistrust of vaccinations and public health interventions can hamper their effectiveness.

b. Outlook

- **Capacity building**: Invest in building the capacity of public health systems to better respond to zoonoses.
- **International collaboration**: Promoting international cooperation to share best practices and resources in the fight against zoonoses.

Regulations and public health policies are essential to prevent and control zoonoses. By setting clear standards, promoting an intersectoral approach and investing in awareness-raising and training, governments can better protect public health and reduce the risks associated with zoonoses. Ongoing collaboration between the various players is necessary to meet the challenges and ensure an effective response in a constantly changing world.

The role of international organizations in the fight against zoonoses

International organizations play a crucial role in the prevention, monitoring and control of zoonoses worldwide. Entities such as the World Health Organization (WHO) and the World Organization for Animal Health (OIE) are at the heart of these efforts. Here's an overview of the key roles played by these organizations.

1. Monitoring and Detection

a. Monitoring systems

- **Data Collection** : WHO and OIE collect and analyze data on the incidence of zoonoses worldwide, providing a global understanding of epidemic trends.
- **Early Warning Systems**: These organizations set up early warning systems to detect disease outbreaks and rapidly inform the countries concerned.

b. Risk assessment

- **Epidemiological Analysis**: They carry out risk assessments to identify potential zoonotic threats and guide appropriate responses.

2. Development of Standards and Guidelines

a. International standards

- **Health Protocols**: WHO develops guidelines for zoonosis management, including recommendations on vaccination, treatment and prevention.
- **Sanitary standards**: The OIE sets international standards for animal health, helping to prevent the spread of zoonotic diseases across borders.

b. Best practices

- **Knowledge sharing**: These organizations facilitate the sharing of best practices and experiences between countries, thus strengthening local capacities.[73]

3. Capacity building

a. Training and education

- **Training programs**: WHO and OIE offer training courses for health professionals, veterinarians and community workers on the prevention and management of zoonoses.
- **Community awareness**: They support awareness campaigns to inform communities about zoonosis risks and prevention measures.

b. Technical support

- **Country Assistance**: These organizations provide technical support to countries to strengthen their public and veterinary health systems, particularly in terms of epidemic surveillance and response.

4. Epidemic Response Coordination

a. Crisis management

- **Concerted responses**: In the event of a zoonoses epidemic, WHO and OIE coordinate international efforts to mobilize resources and provide assistance to affected countries.
- **Response Plans**: They help to draw up emergency response plans, integrating human, animal and environmental health sectors.

[73] Toma B. - The evolution of zoonoses. *Rev. sci. tech. Off. Int. Epiz.* 2000, **19**, 302-309.

b. Multi-sector partnerships

- **Collaboration with other agencies**: WHO and OIE work in close collaboration with other UN agencies, NGOs and governments for an integrated response to zoonoses.

5. Research & Innovation

a. Promoting research

- **Support for research**: These organizations promote research into zoonoses, including the development of new vaccines and treatments.
- **Funding and resources**: They mobilize funding to support innovative research projects in the field of zoonotic diseases.

b. Sharing results

- **Publications and conferences**: WHO and OIE regularly publish reports and organize conferences to share research findings and advances in the field of zoonoses.

International organizations such as the WHO and OIE play an indispensable role in the fight against zoonoses. Through their work in surveillance, standard-setting, capacity-building, coordinating responses and promoting research, they help to protect public health on a global scale. Their collaborative action with countries and other players is essential to meet the growing challenges posed by zoonoses in an interconnected world.

CHAPTER 7: CASE STUDIES

Avian Flu Study: Answers and Lessons Learned

Avian influenza, caused by viruses of the Orthomyxoviridae family, represents a threat to animal and human health. It has caused several epidemics around the world, requiring coordinated responses at different levels. Here is an overview of the responses implemented and the lessons learned.

1. Background and Impact

a. Origins and transmission

- **Influenza A viruses**: Avian flu is mainly caused by strains of influenza A virus, notably H5N1, H7N9 and H5N8, which can spread from birds to humans.
- **Transmission**: Transmission to humans usually occurs through contact with infected birds or their droppings, but cases of human-to-human transmission have also been reported.

b. Health and economic impact

- **Public health**: Human infections can lead to serious illness and a high mortality rate.
- **Economy**: Avian flu epidemics have a major economic impact on poultry farming, resulting in considerable financial losses.[74]

2. Responses to epidemics

a. Monitoring and detection

- **Surveillance systems**: Countries have strengthened their surveillance systems to rapidly detect outbreaks of avian flu in birds and humans.

---

[74] Meslin F.X. - Global aspects of emerging and potential zoonoses: a WHO perspective. *Emerg. Infect. Dis.* 1997, **3**(2), 223-228.

- **Reference laboratories**: Creation of specialized laboratories to diagnose infections and identify viral strains.[75]

b. Control and eradication

- **Sanitary culling**: Preventive culling campaigns for infected poultry have been implemented to limit the spread of the virus.
- **Vaccination**: Development and deployment of poultry vaccines to reduce infection and transmission.

c. Awareness-raising and education

- **Public information**: Awareness campaigns to inform breeders, healthcare workers and the general public about risks and preventive measures.
- **Training for professionals**: training programs for veterinarians and health workers on the management of avian influenza epidemics.

3. International Coordination

a. Worldwide collaboration

- **Partnerships**: WHO, OIE and FAO worked together to coordinate response efforts and provide technical support to affected countries.
- **Early Warning Systems**: Setting up early warning systems to rapidly share information on avian flu outbreaks.

b. Research and development

- **Investment in research**: Encouraging research into avian flu viruses, vaccines and treatments.
- **Data sharing**: creation of databases for sharing research results and epidemiological information.

4. Lessons learned

---

[75] Warrell M.J. and Warrell D.A. - Rabies and other lyssavirus diseases." Lancet, 2004, **363**(9413), 959-969.

a. Importance of surveillance

- **Reinforced surveillance**: Ongoing surveillance is essential for early detection of outbreaks and prevention of epidemics.
- **One Health approach**: Integrating human, animal and environmental health perspectives for more effective surveillance.

b. Epidemic preparedness

- **Contingency plans**: Develop clear, tested contingency plans to respond to avian flu outbreaks.
- **Crisis simulations**: organize simulation exercises to assess the preparedness of public health and veterinary systems.

c. Community awareness

- **Ongoing education**: Community awareness and education are essential to encourage preventive behavior.
- **Involvement of breeders**: Actively involve breeders in vaccination and prevention programs.

d. International collaboration

- **Enhanced partnerships** : Collaboration between countries and international organizations is crucial to managing transnational threats.
- **Sharing best practice**: exchanging ideas and experiences between nations can improve the global response to zoonoses.

To know more

The study of avian influenza highlights the importance of a coordinated and integrated response to manage zoonoses. Lessons learned from these outbreaks underscore the need for enhanced surveillance, effective preparedness, community awareness and international collaboration. By applying these lessons, countries can be better prepared to deal with possible future outbreaks of avian influenza and similar zoonoses.

The Case of COVID-19: Emerging Zoonosis and Crisis Management

The COVID-19 pandemic was an unprecedented global health crisis, caused by the SARS-CoV-2 virus. Considered an emerging zoonosis, the virus highlighted the challenges facing public health, healthcare systems and international cooperation. Here's a look at the key aspects of this crisis and the lessons learned.

1. Origins and transmission

a. Zoonotic origins

- **Animal transmission**: SARS-CoV-2 probably originated in bats and could be transmitted to humans via an intermediate host, underscoring the importance of zoonosis surveillance.
- **Wuhan wet market**: The first cases were linked to a wet market in Wuhan, China, where live animals were sold, highlighting the risks associated with such environments.

b. Transmission modes

- **Human-to-human transmission**: The virus is spread mainly via respiratory droplets, direct contact and sometimes contaminated surfaces.

2. Initial Responses

a. Monitoring and detection

- **Health surveillance systems**: At the start of the pandemic, surveillance systems were activated to detect suspected cases and monitor the spread of the virus.
- **Diagnostic tests**: Rapid development of PCR tests to identify infections, although access has been difficult in several countries.

b. Control measures

- **Confinement and social distancing**: Governments have imposed confinement, travel restrictions and social distancing measures to slow the spread of the virus.
- **Wearing masks**: The recommendation or obligation to wear masks in public spaces has been widely adopted.

3. Crisis management

a. International coordination

- **World Health Organization (WHO)**: WHO played a central role in coordinating the international response, providing guidelines and recommendations.
- **Public-private partnerships**: Collaboration between governments, businesses and NGOs has been crucial to mobilizing resources and sharing information.

b. Vaccine development

- **Speed of development**: Thanks to unprecedented research and funding efforts, several vaccines have been developed and approved in less than a year.
- **Vaccination campaigns**: Mass vaccination campaigns have been launched in many countries to achieve herd immunity.

4. Communication and awareness-raising

a. Raising public awareness

- **Virus information**: Awareness campaigns have been set up to inform the public about symptoms, modes of transmission and preventive measures.
- **Combating misinformation**: Health authorities have had to deal with misinformation and conspiracy theories, requiring extra efforts to provide reliable information.

b. Community involvement

- **Community involvement**: Communities were encouraged to participate in prevention efforts, notably through vaccination initiatives and local awareness campaigns.[76]

5. Lessons learned

a. Importance of surveillance

- **Enhanced surveillance of zoonoses**: The pandemic has highlighted the need to strengthen surveillance of zoonotic diseases and invest in research into viruses of animal origin.

b. Health crisis preparedness

- **Response Plans**: Countries need to develop and test contingency plans to deal with future epidemics, with regular simulations to assess preparedness.

c. International collaboration

- **Working together**: The pandemic has demonstrated the importance of international cooperation in managing health crises and sharing information and resources.

d. Effective communication

- **Communication strategies**: Clear, transparent, evidence-based communication is essential to maintain public confidence and encourage support for public health measures.

The COVID-19 pandemic revealed the vulnerabilities of global healthcare systems in the face of emerging zoonoses. Coordinated responses, the importance of surveillance, rapid vaccine development and effective communication are key lessons to be learned. By incorporating these lessons into future public health

---

[76] Morens D.M., Folkers G.K. and Fauce A.S. - The challenge of emerging and reemerging infectious diseases. Nature, 2004, **430**(6996), 242-249.

strategies, it will be possible to better prepare for such health challenges in the future.

Other Significant Regional Examples of Emerging Zoonoses

Emerging zoonoses represent a global public health challenge, but some regions have experienced notable epidemics that illustrate the risks associated with these diseases. Here are a few significant examples by region.

1. Asia-Pacific

a. Nipah virus (1998, Malaysia)

- **Origin**: Nipah virus was first identified in pig farmers in Malaysia.
- **Transmission**: The virus is spread mainly by direct contact with infected animals, especially bats and pigs.
- **Impact**: The epidemic caused hundreds of human infections and a high mortality rate. It led to strict animal control measures and awareness-raising efforts.

b. H7N9 (2013, China)

- **Origin**: A strain of H7N9 avian flu has been detected in humans, linked to infected poultry.
- **Transmission**: Human transmission has been limited, but severe cases have been reported.
- **Impact**: Poultry vaccination campaigns and restrictions on live poultry markets have been implemented to control the spread.

2. Africa

a. Ebola (2014-2016, West Africa)

- **Origin**: The Ebola virus was identified in bats and spread to humans through contact with the bodily fluids of infected animals.
- **Transmission**: Human-to-human transmission has been facilitated by cultural practices such as funerals.

- **Impact**: Over 11,000 deaths were recorded. The response included vaccination campaigns, contact tracing and awareness-raising efforts.

b. Lassa fever (Nigeria)

- **Origin**: Lassa fever is caused by the Lassa virus, transmitted by rodents.
- **Transmission**: Human transmission occurs through contact with the excrement or urine of infected rodents.
- **Impact**: Lassa fever is endemic in certain regions, leading to seasonal epidemics. Awareness-raising and vaccination programs are underway.

3. Americas

a. Zika virus (2015-2016, Latin America)

- **Origin**: The Zika virus, transmitted by mosquitoes, has caused massive epidemics, particularly in Brazil.
- **Transmission**: Transmission is mainly by Aedes mosquito bites, but sexual transmission has also been reported.
- **Impact**: The epidemic was associated with birth defects, notably microcephaly. It required a rapid public health response, including vector control campaigns.

b. Rage (State of Texas, USA)

- **Origin**: Rabies is a viral zoonosis transmitted by the saliva of infected animals.
- **Transmission**: Cases of rabies are often linked to bites from wild or domestic animals.
- **Impact**: Vaccination of domestic animals and awareness campaigns have been put in place to reduce human rabies cases.

4. Europe

a. Lyme disease (Europe)

- **Origin**: Caused by the Borrelia bacterium, Lyme disease is transmitted by ticks.
- **Transmission**: Transmission occurs mainly through the bites of infected ticks.

- **Impact**: Cases of Lyme disease have increased in Europe, necessitating awareness-raising efforts and tick population management programs.

b. Q fever (Europe)

- **Origin**: Caused by the bacterium Coxiella burnetii, Q fever is often associated with farm animals such as sheep and goats.
- **Transmission**: Transmission occurs through inhalation of contaminated airborne particles.
- **Impact**: Epidemics have been reported in Europe, leading to increases in human cases. Farm control measures and animal vaccination campaigns have been implemented.

These regional examples illustrate the diversity of emerging zoonoses and the responses required to control them. Surveillance, awareness-raising, vaccination and international coordination are essential elements in preventing and managing zoonosis epidemics. Each region needs to adapt its strategies to the specific risks and local contexts in order to improve public health and protect communities.

CHAPTER 8: FUTURE PROSPECTS

8.1. Innovations in Zoonoses Research

Research into zoonoses has seen significant advances, aided by technological and methodological innovations. These innovations are essential to better understand, prevent and control diseases of animal origin that affect human health. Here's an overview of the main innovations in this field.

1.1 Genetic Sequencing Technology

a. Next-generation sequencing (NGS)

- **Description**: NGS makes it possible to sequence entire viral and bacterial genomes rapidly and cost-effectively.
- **Impact**: This technology has been crucial in identifying and tracking strains of zoonotic pathogens, such as SARS-CoV-2, in real time, facilitating rapid responses to epidemics.

b. Phylogenetic analysis

- **Description**: Phylogenetic tools can be used to analyze the evolutionary relationships between different strains of pathogens.
- **Impact**: This helps to understand transmission between animals and humans, as well as the evolution of pathogens.[77]

8.1.2. Epidemiological modeling

[77] cf. Espinosa R., N .Gaidet and N.Treich (2020) " Il faut prendre en considération le rôle de la consommation de viande et l'élevage intensif dans ces nouvelles épidémies ". Tribune TSE (Le Monde 20/3/2020) .Leroy P., Requillart V. and L.G.Soler (2017), " Entre préservation de l'environnement et santé, une analyse coût-bénéfice des recommandations alimentaires ", INRA, Sciences sociales N°5/2016

a. Mathematical models

- **Description** : Mathematical models can be used to simulate the spread of zoonoses and assess the impact of interventions.
- **Impact**: These models help predict outbreaks and plan effective control strategies.

b. Big Data and Data Analysis

- **Description**: The integration of large quantities of data from various sources (public health, agriculture, environment) enables a more in-depth analysis of zoonoses.
- **Impact**: These analyses improve our understanding of risk factors and transmission patterns.

3. Vaccines and therapies

a. Messenger RNA vaccines

- **Description**: mRNA vaccines, such as those developed for COVID-19, represent a promising innovation in the prevention of zoonoses.
- **Impact**: This technology enables a rapid, adaptable response to new pathogens, with potential applications for zoonotic diseases.

b. Veterinary vaccines

- **Description**: Vaccines for livestock and companion animals are being developed to prevent the transmission of zoonoses such as rabies and certain strains of avian flu.
- **Impact**: Vaccinating animals helps reduce the risk of human infection.

4. Monitoring and detection

a. Intelligent Monitoring Systems

- **Description**: The use of sensors, drones and Internet of Things (IoT) technologies to monitor animal populations and detect emerging epidemics.

- **Impact**: These systems enable early detection and rapid response to zoonotic threats.

b. Quick Diagnostics

- **Description**: Development of rapid, sensitive diagnostic tests to detect zoonoses in animals and humans.
- **Impact**: Faster diagnosis means more effective containment of infection outbreaks.

5. One Health approach

a. Multi-sector integration

- **Description**: Research promotes a One Health approach, linking human, animal and environmental health.
- **Impact**: This leads to a better understanding of the complex interactions between these fields and contributes to integrated prevention strategies.

b. Interdisciplinary collaboration

- **Description**: Encouraging collaboration between researchers, veterinarians, physicians and ecologists to take a holistic approach to zoonoses.
- **Impact**: This collaboration enriches knowledge and improves responses to epidemics.

Innovations in zoonoses research offer new perspectives for understanding and controlling these diseases. Thanks to technological advances in sequencing, modeling, vaccination and surveillance, it is possible to significantly improve the prevention and management of zoonoses. Integrating these innovations into a One Health approach is crucial to meeting future challenges and protecting global public health.

The importance of One Health

The One Health concept is based on the idea that human, animal and environmental health are interconnected. This integrated approach is essential for tackling global health challenges, including zoonoses, pandemics and environmental problems. Here are the main reasons why One Health is crucial.

1. Zoonotic Disease Prevention

a. Integrated monitoring

- **Early detection**: Combined monitoring of human, animal and environmental populations enables early detection of zoonotic disease outbreaks.
- **Data sharing**: A collaborative approach encourages the sharing of information between vets, doctors and ecologists, boosting responsiveness to threats.

b. Harm reduction

- **Vector control**: By tackling the environmental factors that favor disease transmission, we can reduce the risk of epidemics.
- **Animal Vaccination**: Vaccinating domestic and farm animals helps protect human health by reducing the transmission of zoonoses.

2. Pandemic response

a. Multisectoral approach

- **Interdisciplinary collaboration**: One Health encourages cooperation between different sectors, such as public health, agriculture and the environment, for a coordinated response to pandemics.
- **Crisis management**: By integrating knowledge and resources from different fields, the response to health crises such as COVID-19 is more effective.

b. Capacity building

- **Preparedness plans**: One Health enables the development of pandemic preparedness plans that take into account the complex interactions between the various healthcare fields.

3. Food safety

a. Sustainable production

- **Responsible animal husbandry**: Promoting sustainable agricultural practices and responsible animal husbandry contributes to food safety while minimizing health risks.
- **Disease control**: An integrated approach helps to control animal diseases that can affect the food chain and human health.

b. Food quality

- **Food Chain Monitoring**: One Health monitors the food chain for contaminants and pathogens, ensuring safe food.

4. Environmental protection

a. Ecosystem conservation

- **Biodiversity**: Preserving biodiversity is essential to maintaining healthy ecosystems, which in turn contributes to human and animal health.
- **Ecological balance**: A One Health approach helps to understand how environmental disturbances can promote the emergence of disease.

b. Climate change

- **Adaptation and resilience**: By integrating the impacts of climate change on health, One Health helps develop adaptation strategies to reduce future health risks.

5. Education and awareness

a. Professional training

- **Interdisciplinary education**: Educating health professionals, veterinarians and ecologists about the interconnections between their fields is essential for an effective response.
- **Raising public awareness**: Informing the general public about the links between human, animal and environmental health encourages preventive behavior.

b. Community involvement

- **Citizen participation**: Encouraging communities to get involved in public health initiatives strengthens resilience in the face of health threats.

The One Health approach is essential to meeting the complex challenges of global health. By recognizing the interconnection between human, animal and environmental health, this approach promotes an integrated and effective response to zoonoses, pandemics and environmental problems. By investing in a One Health strategy, countries can improve public health, enhance food security and protect ecosystems, thereby contributing to a healthier, more sustainable future for all.

Recommendations for a Better Public Health Policy

The development of effective public health policies is essential to improving the health of populations and responding to emerging health challenges. Here are some key recommendations for strengthening public health policies.

1. Strengthening surveillance and detection

- **Integrated Surveillance Systems**: Establish surveillance systems that integrate human, animal and environmental health to rapidly detect epidemics and zoonoses.
- **Detection technologies**: Investing in advanced technologies, such as genetic sequencing and data analysis, to improve the speed and accuracy of diagnosis.

2. Promoting the One Health approach

- **Intersectoral Collaboration**: Promoting cooperation between the public health, agriculture, environment and research sectors for a coordinated response to health threats.
- **Interdisciplinary training**: Integrating One Health education into training programs for healthcare professionals, veterinarians and scientists.

3. Strengthening response capabilities

- **Contingency plans**: Develop and test robust contingency plans to deal with epidemics, with clear protocols for detection, response and communication.
- **Simulation exercises**: Organize regular simulations and exercises to assess the readiness of public health systems.

4. Increasing access to healthcare

- **Resilient Health Systems**: Investing in sustainable, accessible healthcare infrastructure, particularly in rural and disadvantaged areas.
- **Expanding health coverage**: Promoting universal access to healthcare for all, by reducing financial and geographical barriers.

5. Education and awareness

- **Education campaigns**: Implement awareness campaigns to inform the public about health risks, disease prevention and the importance of vaccination.
- **Community involvement**: Encouraging community participation in the design and implementation of public health programs.[78]

6. Investing in Research and Innovation

- **Research funding**: Increase funding for research into zoonoses, emerging diseases and innovative public health solutions.
- **Public-Private Partnerships**: Encourage collaboration between the public sector, private companies and academic institutions to develop new technologies and approaches.

7. Policy Evaluation and Monitoring

- **Evaluation mechanisms**: Set up evaluation systems to measure the effectiveness of public health policies and adjust strategies accordingly.
- **Transparency and Accountability**: Promoting transparency in the communication of results and

[78] According to S.Morand. Answers to "Libération" (26/3/2020)

decisions, thereby strengthening public confidence in healthcare institutions.

8. International Coordination

- **Global collaboration**: Working with international organizations, such as the WHO and OIE, to share information, resources and best practices.
- **Health Crisis Response**: Establish mechanisms for rapid response to health crises on a global scale, incorporating lessons learned from past experience.

By implementing these recommendations, governments and public health institutions can create more effective and resilient policies, capable of addressing current and future health challenges. An integrated and collaborative approach is essential to protect the health of populations and improve collective well-being.

Call to action for decision-makers and healthcare professionals

In the face of growing public health challenges, including emerging zoonoses, pandemics and environmental problems, it is crucial that decision-makers and healthcare professionals take immediate and coordinated action. Here's a call to action structured into several key points.

1. Strengthening healthcare systems

- **Investing in infrastructure**: Allocate sufficient resources to modernize and strengthen healthcare infrastructure, ensuring that it is accessible to all populations, particularly in rural and disadvantaged areas.
- **Training healthcare personnel**: Implement ongoing training programs for healthcare professionals, to prepare them to manage epidemics and adopt a One Health approach.

2. Promoting the One Health approach

- **Encourage Intersectoral Collaboration**: Create collaborative platforms between the human, animal and environmental health sectors to share data and coordinate responses to health threats.

- **Raising awareness of Global Health**: Integrating the One Health concept into educational programs for healthcare professionals, emphasizing the interconnection between different disciplines.

3. Improving Monitoring and Detection

- **Establish Effective Surveillance Systems**: Set up robust surveillance systems to rapidly detect epidemics and zoonoses, using cutting-edge technologies such as genetic sequencing.
- **Promoting public health research**: investing in research to develop rapid, accurate diagnostic tools, as well as innovative treatments and vaccines.

4. Strengthen Communication and Education

- **Launch Awareness Campaigns**: Organize educational campaigns on the importance of disease prevention, vaccination and public health behaviors.
- **Involving communities**: Encourage the participation of communities in the design and implementation of health programs, by listening to their needs and concerns.

5. Promoting inclusive healthcare policies

- **Ensuring Health Equity**: Developing policies that guarantee equitable access to healthcare, taking into account vulnerable and marginalized populations.
- **Evaluate and adjust policies**: Put in place evaluation mechanisms to measure the impact of public health policies and adjust strategies according to the results obtained.

6. Strengthening international coordination

- **Collaborate with Global Organizations**: Work closely with international organizations, such as the WHO and OIE, to share information and coordinate efforts to respond to health crises.

- **Participate in Global Initiatives**: Get involved in international initiatives aimed at preventing the emergence of zoonoses and strengthening the resilience of healthcare systems.

Decision-makers and healthcare professionals play a crucial role in protecting public health and preventing health crises. By taking immediate and coordinated action, you can help build more resilient and equitable healthcare systems, capable of meeting tomorrow's challenges. A collective commitment to the One Health approach and cross-sector collaboration are essential to ensure a healthy and sustainable future for all communities. Together, let's act now for a healthier world!

Appendix

Glossary of Technical Terms

Here's a glossary of technical terms commonly used in the field of public health, zoonoses and the One Health approach.

1. Zoonosis

Disease or infection that spreads from animals to humans. Examples include rabies, avian flu and the Ebola virus.

2. One Health

An integrated approach that recognizes the interconnection between human, animal and environmental health, with the aim of improving overall health.

3. Epidemiological surveillance

The process of collecting, analyzing and interpreting health data to detect and respond to epidemics and diseases.

4. Genetic sequencing

A technique for determining the order of bases in DNA or RNA, used to identify pathogens and track their evolution.

5. Vaccine

Biological preparation administered to induce an immune response and protect against an infectious disease.

6. Diagnostics

The process of determining the nature of a disease or condition by examining symptoms and medical tests.

7. Epidemic

Rapid increase in the number of cases of a disease in a given population or region over a specific period.

8. Pandemic

An epidemic that spreads over several countries or continents, affecting large numbers of people. COVID-19 is a recent example.

9. Vector

Living organism that transmits a pathogen from one host to another, such as mosquitoes for the Zika virus or malaria.

10. Health risk

Probability that an event or exposure will lead to adverse effects on human health.

11. Health care system

A set of organizations, institutions and resources that provide health services to a population.

12. Health Equity

The principle that all individuals should have equal access to healthcare, regardless of their socio-economic status.

13. Antigen

Substance that provokes an immune response, often used in vaccine development.

14. Collective immunity

Indirect protection of a population against a disease when enough individuals are immune, thus reducing transmission.

15. Infection

Invasion and multiplication of pathogenic micro-organisms in the body, which can cause disease.

16. Pathogen

Micro-organism (virus, bacterium, fungus or parasite) capable of causing disease.

17. Risk assessment

The process of identifying and analyzing potential health hazards in order to make informed risk management decisions.

18. Ecosystem

System formed by the interaction of living organisms and their environment, influencing overall health.

19. Preventive medicine

An approach that aims to prevent disease rather than treat it, through vaccinations, screening and health promotion.

20. Resilient Health System

A system capable of adapting and responding effectively to health crises while maintaining essential health services.

This glossary provides a basis for understanding the technical terms associated with public health and zoonoses. A clear understanding of these terms is essential for decision-makers, healthcare professionals and the general public to better grasp global health issues.

How to prevent Zoonoses

To prevent zoonoses, it's essential to adopt a multifaceted approach involving prevention, education and awareness-raising measures. Here are some key recommendations:

1. Hygiene and Sanitary Practices

- **Hand washing**: Wash hands regularly, especially after handling animals or coming into contact with potentially contaminated surfaces.

- **Avoiding contact with sick animals**: Limit interaction with animals showing signs of illness.[79]

2. Food safety

- **Proper cooking**: Cook meat, fish and eggs at safe temperatures to kill pathogens.
- **Avoid raw foods**: Limit consumption of raw or unpasteurized meat, seafood and dairy products.

3. Vector control

- **Insect control**: Use insecticides and repellents to control mosquito and tick populations.
- **Waste disposal**: Eliminate waste and sources of stagnant water to reduce vector habitats.

4. Education and awareness

- **Awareness programs**: Promote educational campaigns on zoonoses and their modes of transmission.
- **Breeder awareness**: Train breeders in best animal management practices to prevent infections.

5. Monitoring and Early Detection

- **Disease surveillance**: set up surveillance systems to rapidly detect epidemics in animals and humans.
- **Suspicious Case Reporting**: Encourage reporting of animal and human diseases.

6. Vaccination

- **Animal Vaccination**: Vaccinate pets and farm animals against zoonotic diseases.

---

[79] Zucca, P. 2020. The zoonosecene: the new geological epoch of intensive breeding, of wildlife trade, of antibiotic resistance and of pandemic diseases, following the anthropocene. *Platinum.* 11:114. doi: 10.13140/RG.2.2.16949.50408/1 3. Friend, M. 2006. *Disease Emergence and*

- **Human vaccination**: Follow vaccination recommendations for people at risk.[80]

7. Sound Environmental Practices

- **Sustainable Ecosystem Management**: Protecting natural habitats and promoting biodiversity to reduce the risk of new zoonoses emerging.
- **Avoiding poaching**: Protecting wildlife to prevent the transmission of diseases to humans.[81]

General conclusion on Zoonoses

Zoonoses represent a major public health issue, linking human, animal and environmental health in a complex and dynamic framework. Global population growth, urbanization and environmental change exacerbate the risks associated with these transmissible infections.

1. Importance of Monitoring and Prevention

Preventing zoonoses requires close monitoring of epidemics, as well as interdisciplinary collaboration between health professionals, veterinarians and ecologists. Effective surveillance systems enable us to detect emerging diseases early and intervene before they become public health crises.

2. Awareness and education

Community awareness and education on modes of transmission, symptoms and preventive measures are essential. By informing the public about zoonoses, we can reduce risk behaviors and promote preventive practices.

3. Sustainable Practices

---

[80] Friend, M. 2006. *Disease Emergence and Resurgence: The Wildlife-Human*
Connection. Vol. 1285. Reston, VA: US department of the Interior, US Geological Survey. doi: 10.3133/cir1285

[81] De Kruif, P. 1926. *Microbe Hunter.* New York, NY: Harcourt Brace

The adoption of sustainable agricultural practices and the responsible management of natural resources are crucial to minimizing the risk of new zoonoses emerging. Protecting biodiversity and ecosystems also contributes to reducing contact between humans and pathogens.

4. One Health" approach

The "One Health" approach emphasizes the interconnection between human, animal and environmental health. By integrating this perspective, we can better anticipate and respond to the challenges posed by zoonoses, promoting global and sustainable solutions.

Final conclusion

Ultimately, the fight against zoonoses requires a collective commitment at all levels of society. By working together to improve surveillance, strengthen education, adopt sustainable practices and promote an integrated approach to health, we can better protect individuals, communities and our planet from the threats posed by zoonoses. Everyone's health depends on our ability to understand and manage these diseases proactively.

Preventing zoonoses requires cooperation between human, animal and environmental health professionals. By adopting these measures, we can reduce the risk of infection and protect public health in the long term.

BIBLIOGRAPHY

Acha P.N., Szyfres B., 2005. *Zoonoses and communicable diseases common to man and animals*, OIE.

Artaud H. *et al.*, 2019. *Museum Manifesto. Humans and other animals.* Reliefs/MNHN, https://www.mnhn.fr/fr/explorez/actualites/ manifest-museum-humans-other-animals.

Barnouin J., Sache Y., 2010. *Emerging diseases. Epidemiology in plants, animals and humans*. Editions Qu..

Blanc S., Boetsch G., Hossaert-McKey M., Renaud F., 2017. *Health ecology*, https://www.cnrs.fr/fr/ecologie-de-la-sante-pour-unenouvelle- read-my-health.

Duvallet G., Fontenille D., Robert V., 2017. *Medical and veterinary entomology*. IRD Editions, Editions Qu..

Guegan J.-F., Choisy M., 2008. *Introduction to the integrative epidemiology of infectious and parasitic diseases*. De Boeck Superieur.

Leport C., Guegan J.-F., 2011. *Emerging infectious diseases: status and outlook*. La Documentation française, https://www. Vie publique.fr/rapport/31962-les-maladies-infectieuses-emergentesetat- de-la-situation et-perspecti.

Report by the Foundation for Biodiversity Research (FRB), 2020. *Mobilisation de la FRB par les pouvoirs publics français sur les liens entre Covid-19 et biodiversité*,https://www.fondationbiodiversite.fr/wp-content/uploads/2020/05/Mobilisation-FRBCovid- 19-15-05-2020-1.pdf.

Report of the "Intergovernmental Science-Policy Platform on Biodiversity and Ecosystem Services" (IPBES) seminar on Escaping the Era of Pandemics, 2020, https://ipbes.net/pandemics. Vittecoq M., Roche B., Prugnolle F., Renaud F., Thomas F., 2015. *Les maladies infectieuses*. De Boeck-Solal.

Morand S., 2016. *The next plague. A global history of societies and their epidemics.* Editions Fayard.
[1] Morand S., 2020. *Man, wildlife and the plague.* Editions Fayard.
Morand S., Figuie M., 2016. *Emerging infectious diseases. Risques et enjeux de société.* Editions Qu..

Morand S., Lajaunie C., 2018. *Biodiversity and health. Links between living organisms, ecosystems and societies.* ISTE/Elsevier.

Morand S., Moutou F., Richomme C., 2014. *Faune sauvage, biodiversité et santé, quels défis?* Editions Qu..

Moutou F., 2020. *Epidemics, animals and people.* Editions Le Pommier.

World Health Organization (WHO). WHO | Zoonoses and the Environment [Internet]. WHO. World Health Organization; 2020 [cited26 Apr2020]. Available from: https://www.who.int/foodsafety/areas_work/zoonose/fr/

HubálekZ. Emerging Human Infectious Diseases: Anthroponoses, Zoonoses, and Sapronoses-Volume 9, Number 3-March 2003 -Emerging Infectious Diseases journal CDC. 2003 [cited26 Apr2020];9(3). Available from: https://wwwnc.cdc.gov/eid/article/9/3/02-0208_article

Lowe A-M. Bulletin de l'Observatoire multipartite québécois sur les zoonoses et l'adaptation aux changements climatiques, Volume1

[Internet]. INSPQ. [cited 26 Apr2020]. Available from: https://www.inspq.qc.ca/bulletin-de-l-observatoire-multipartite-quebecois-sur-les-zoonoses-et-l-adaptation-aux-changements-climatiques/janvier-2016

Larousse É. Definitions: prion -Dictionnaire de français Larousse [Internet]. [cited 26 Apr2020]. Available from: https://www.larousse.fr/dictionnaires/francais/prion/63977

PrusinerSB. Novelproteinaceousinfectiousparticlescause scrapie. Science. 9 avr1982;216(4542):136-44.

Larousse É. Definitions: parasite -Dictionnaire de français Larousse [Internet]. [cited 26 Apr2020]. Available from: https://www.larousse.fr/dictionnaires/francais/parasite/58023

BourgeadeA, DavoustB, GallaisH. FROM ANIMAL DISEASES TO HUMAN INFECTIONS. Médecine d'Afrique Noire. 1992;39(3):6.

Larousse É. Definitions: parasite -Dictionnaire de français Larousse [Internet]. [cited 26 Apr2020]. Available from: https://www.larousse.fr/dictionnaires/francais/parasite/58023

Zoonotic Diseases | One Health | CDC [Internet]. 2020 [cited 26 Apr2020]. Available from: https://www.cdc.gov/onehealth/basics/zoonotic-diseases.html

World Organisation for Animal Health (OIE). One health: OIE - World Organisation for Animal Health [Internet]. 2020 [cited 26 Apr2020]. Available from: https://www.oie.int/fr/pour-les-medias/une-seule-sante/

[1] One Health initiative. One Health Initiative -One World One Medicine One Health [Internet]. Mission Statement. [cited 26 Apr2020]. Available from: http://www.onehealthinitiative.com/mission.php

[1] Han BA, Kramer AM, Drake JM. Global Patterns of Zoonotic Disease in Mammals. Trends in Parasitology. 1 Jul2016;32(7):565-77.

Van den Berg T. One health paradigm to foster population health [Internet]. BiomedCentral. 2020 [cited 26 Apr2020]. Available from: https://www.biomedcentral.com/collections/OneHealth

KeesingF, Belden LK, DaszakP, Dobson A, Harvell CD, Holt RD, et al. Impacts of biodiversity on the emergence and transmission of infectious diseases. Nature. déc2010;468(7324):647-52.

WoldehannaS, ZimickiS. An expanded One Health model: Integrating social science and One Health to inform study of the human-animal interface. Social Science & Medicine. March 1, 2015;129:87-95.

KeesingF, Belden LK, DaszakP, Dobson A, Harvell CD, Holt RD, et al. Impacts of biodiversity on the emergence and transmission of infectious diseases. Nature. déc2010;468(7324):647-52.

Barbosa Costa G, Gilbert A, Monroe B, Blanton J, NgamNgamS, RecuencoS, et al. The influence of poverty and rabies knowledge on healthcare seeking behaviors and dog ownership, Cameroon. PLoSOne [Internet]. Jun 21, 2018 [cited 29 Apr2020];13(6). Available from: https://www.ncbi.nlm.nih.gov/pmc/articles/PMC6013156/
CleavelandS, Sharp J, Abela-Ridder B, Allan KJ, BuzaJ, Crump JA, et al. One Health contributions towards more effective and equitable approaches to health in low-and middle-income countries. Philos Trans R Soc LondB BiolSci[Internet]. 19Jul2017 [cited 27 Apr2020];372(1725). Available from: https://www.ncbi.nlm.nih.gov/pmc/articles/PMC5468693/

Rahman MHAA, HaironSM, HamatRA, JamaluddinTZMT, ShafeiMN, Idris N, et al. LeptospirosisHealthIntervention Module Effecton Knowledge, Attitude, Belief, and Practice amongWetMarketWorkersin NortheasternMalaysia: An Intervention Study. Int J Environ ResPublic Health[Internet]. jul2018 [cited 2020 Jun 24];15(7). Available from: https://www.ncbi.nlm.nih.gov/pmc/articles/PMC6069487/

[1] [1] (M.) SAVEY, Commentaire de l'Agence française de sécurité sanitaire des aliments (AFSSA) In La maîtrise des maladies infectieuses, RST n° 24, Académie des sciences, 385- 387, EDP Sciences, 2006.

[2] (V.) DEUBEL, emerging viruses In La maîtrise des maladies infectieuses, RST n° 24, Académie des sciences, 69-87, EDP Sciences, 2006.

[4] (I.T.) EVANS, (E.G.) SMITH, (A.) BANERJEE & coll, Cluster of human tuberculosis caused by Mycobacterium bovis: Evidence for person-to-person transmission in the UK, Lancet, 2007, 369, 1270-1276.

[3] AFSSA, Rapport sur l'évaluation du risque d'apparition et de développement de maladies animales compte tenu d'un éventuel réchauffement climatique, 78 p., 2005.

[5] (J.) COLLINGE & (A.R.) CLARKE, A general model of prion strains and their pathogenecity, Science, 2007, 318, 930-936.

(N.D.) WOLFE, (C.P.) DUNAVAN & (J.) DIAMOND, origins of major human infectious diseases, Nature, 447, 279-283, 2007.

[6] AFSSA - Report on H5N1 highly pathogenic avian influenza of Asian origin, 212 p., 2008 (forthcoming).

(N.D.) WOLFE, (C.P.) DUNAVAN & (J.) DIAMOND, origins of major human infectious diseases, Nature, 447, 279-283, 2007.

(N.D.) WOLFE, (C.P.) DUNAVAN & (J.) DIAMOND, origins of major human infectious diseases, Nature, 447, 279-283, 2007.
Canadian Food Inspection Agency. (2003b). Rapport annuel, Questionnaire FAO/ OIE/ OMS - 2003, Canada, Report submitted to the Office International des Épizooties. Available February 22, 2006 at www.inspection.gc.ca/francais/anima/surv/ 2003oief. shtml

Canadian Food Inspection Agency. (2005). Hantavirus pulmonary syndrome. Accessed October 18, 2005 at www.inspection.gc.ca/francais/anima/heasan/disemala/ hanta/hantafsf.shtml

Canadian Food Inspection Agency. (2003a). Rabies. Accessed November 2, 2005 at www.inspection.gc.ca/ english/anima/heasan/disemala/rabrag/rabragfsf.shtml

Public Health Agency of Canada (2006). Notifiable diseases online - Rabies. Accessed February 22, 2006 at http://dsol-smed.phac aspc.gc.ca/dsol-smed/ ndis/disease2/ rabi_e.html

Public Health Agency of Canada (2005a). Disease Information - Malaria. Accessed October 20, 2005 at www. phac-aspc.gc.ca/tmp-pmv/info/pal_mal_e.html

Public Health Agency of Canada (2005b). News briefs for infectious diseases. Available November 11, 2005 at www.phac-aspc.gc.ca/bid bmi/dsddsm/ nb-ab/index_e. html

Public Health Agency of Canada (2005d). Notifiable diseases online. Available November 3, 2005 at http://dsol-smed.phac-aspc.gc.ca/dsol smed/ndis/ list_f. html#tab2<

Bouden M., Moulin, B., Gosselin, P., Back, C., Doyon, B., Gingras, D. & Lebel, G. (2005). Geo-simulation of West Nile virus infection as a function of climate: a public health risk management tool. C-CIARN Conference 2005. Adapting to Climate Change in Canada 2005: Understanding the Risks and Building Capacity. Montreal. May 4-7, 2005.

Binder S., A M Levitt, and J M Hughes (1999). Preventing emerging infectious diseases as we enter the 21st century: CDC's strategy. Public Health Rep. Mar-Apr; 114(2): 130- 134.

Center for Disease Control and Prevention. (2004). The Impact of Malaria, a Leading Cause of Death Worldwide. Accessed February 27, 2006 at www.cdc.gov/malaria/ impact/index.htm

Government of Quebec (2005a). An Act respecting medical laboratories, the preservation of organs, tissues, gametes and embryos and the disposal of cadavers. Accessible November 12, 2005 at www2.publicationsduquebec.gouv.qc.ca/ dynamicSearch/telecharge. php?type=2&file=/ L_0_2/L0_2.html

Giguère, M. (2005). The health impacts of heat waves and the urban heat island effect: A review of current adaptation initiatives in Quebec. Essay submitted for Master's degree in Environment, Université de Sherbrooke, 57 pages and appendices.

Héma-Québec (2005b). Info, Newsletter for volunteers, blood donors and partners. Available February 28, 2006 at www.hema-quebec.qc.ca/media/ english/publications/ infohq_aut05eng.pdf

Haines A., McMichael, A.J. & Epstein, P.R. (2000). Environment and health: 2. Global climate change and health. JAMC;163(6):729-34.

MacLean, J.D., Demers, A.-M., Ndao, M., Kokoskin, E., Ward, B.J. & Gyorkos, T.W. (2004). Malaria epidemics and surveillance systems in Canada. Emerg Infect Dis;10 (7) : 1195- 1201.

Ministère de l'Agriculture, des Pêcheries et de l'Alimentation du Québec (2006a). Surveillance de la santé animale. Available online June 28, 2006 at www.mapaq.gouv.qc.ca/ Fr/Productions/ santeanimale/surveillance/

Ministère de l'Agriculture, des Pêcheries et de l'Alimentation du Québec (2006b). Avian influenza. Available online June 28, 2006 at www.mapaq.gouv.qc.ca/Fr/Productions/ santeanimale/surveillance/maladies animales/grippeaviaire

Ogden, N.H., Maarouf, A., Barker, I.K., Bigras-Poulin, M., Lindsay, L.R., Morshed, M.G.,
O'Callaghan, C.J., Ramay, F., Waltner-Toews, D., Charron, D.F. Climate change and the potential for range expansion of the Lyme disease vector Ixodes scapularis in Canada.
Int J Parasitol. 2006 Jan;36(1):63-70.
Health Canada (2005). Your Health and a Changing Climate: Newsletter.
Accessible August 25, 2005 at www.c-ciarn.ca/health/app/filerepository/ 348DC2838BCB 498DB86828FA12122713.pdf

Pollution probe (2004). Primer on climate change and human health. Accessible August 25, 2005 at www.pollution probe.org/Reports/climatechange primer(en).pdf

Badin de Montjoye Th., Thorel M.F. and Garin-Bastuji B. - Trends in bovine tuberculosis in France: 2002 review and outlook. *Bull. GTV*, 2004, **23**, 311- 314.

Acha P.N. and Szyfres B. - Zoonoses and communicable diseases common to man and animals (Second edition). Office International des Epizooties, 1989, 1063p.

Chomel B. - Emerging bacterial zoonoses. *Point Vét*, 2000, **31**, 195- 202.

Bénet J.J. and Haddad N. - Dangers, risks and prevention of zoonoses transmitted to humans by dog and cat bites. *Le Nouveau Praticien Vétérinaire*, 2004, **18**, 21-25.

Hantz S. and Darde M.L. - How to prevent the risks of zoonosis for the immunocompromised subject. *Le nouveau praticien vétérinaire*, 2004, **18**, 41-43.

Hahn B.H., Shaw G.M., De Cock K.M. and Sharp P.M. - AIDS as a zoonosis: scientific and public health implications. *Science*, 2000, **287**(5453), 607-614.

Hubalek Z. - Emerging human infectious diseases: anthroponoses, zoonoses, and sapronoses. *Emerg. Infect. Dis*. 2003; **9**(3); 403-404.

Haydon D.T., Cleaveland S., Taylor L.H. and Laurenson - Identifying reservoirs of infection: a conceptual and practical challenge. *Emerg. Infect. Dis*. 2002, **8**(12), 1468-1473.

Toma B. - The evolution of zoonoses. *Rev. sci. tech. Off. Int. Epiz*. 2000, **19**, 302-309.
Meslin F.X. - Global aspects of emerging and potential zoonoses: a WHO perspective. *Emerg. Infect. Dis.* 1997, **3**(2), 223-228.

Warrell M.J. and Warrell D.A. - Rabies and other lyssavirus diseases." Lancet, 2004, **363**(9413), 959-969.

Morens D.M., Folkers G.K. and Fauce A.S. - The challenge of emerging and reemerging infectious diseases. Nature, 2004, **430**(6996), 242-249.

cf. Espinosa R., N .Gaidet and N.Treich (2020) " Il faut prendre en considération le rôle de la consommation de viande et l'élevage intensif dans ces nouvelles épidémies ". Tribune TSE (Le Monde 20/3/2020) .Leroy P., Requillart V. and L.G.Soler (2017), " Entre préservation de l'environnement et santé, une analyse coût-bénéfice des recommandations alimentaires ", INRA, Sciences sociales N°5/2016

According to S.Morand. Answers to "Libération" (26/3/2020)

Zucca, P. 2020. The zoonosecene: the new geological epoch of intensive breeding, of wildlife trade, of antibiotic resistance and of pandemic diseases, following the anthropocene. *Platinum.* 11:114. doi: 10.13140/RG.2.2.16949.50408/1 3. Friend, M. 2006. *Disease Emergence and*

Friend, M. 2006. *Disease Emergence and Resurgence: The Wildlife-Human Connection.* Vol. 1285. Reston, VA: US department of the Interior, US Geological Survey. doi: 10.3133/cir1285

De Kruif, P. 1926. *Microbe Hunter.* New York, NY: Harcourt Brace

TABLE OF CONTENTS

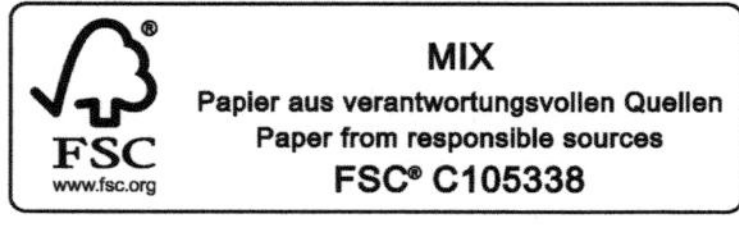

Printed by Books on Demand GmbH, Norderstedt / Germany